"How can a baby's little body inhabit so much space in our homes and in our hearts? *Baby Bare* shows us how we can help our infant fully live into their own bodies so that they build the foundation for a happy and balanced life. . . . This book has wisdom and depth and yet is joyful and fun. It will leave you with a feeling like, 'I can do this!'"

—Kim John Payne, M.Ed, author of the best-selling *Simplicity Parenting* and also *Beyond Winning* and *The Soul of Discipline*

"This is a truly wonderful and greatly needed book for new parents. As a behavioral and developmental pediatrician for the past thirty years, I know how crucial early movement is for creating the structures of the brain that allow for the higher capacities of learning and imaginative thinking. Phonetic-based reading and simultaneous inner mental picturing depend on these neurological pathways being fully developed by the joy-filled, rhythmic movements in infancy and early childhood that are beautifully illustrated in this book."

—Susan R. Johnson, MD, FAAP

"*Baby Bare* is a must-read for parents, grandparents, daycare providers, and early-childhood educators. This beautifully illustrated and easy to understand book, based on neuroscience, offers sound advice for caregivers who want to nurture children to have strong brains, bodies, and social intelligence. Stephanie Johnson clearly explains all the ways that movement and a loving adult are the foundation."

—Anne Green Gilbert, educator, author, and developer of *BrainDance*

"A treasure store of information and strategies for parents and early childhood professionals. . . . This remarkable book is a rare synthesis and visionary thinking with practicality that will immediately benefit parents, early childhood professionals, and most important, the children."

—Deborah Young, Ed. S, PhD, professor contemplative education, early childhood education, Naropa University

"I recommend [*Baby Bare*] highly and plan to share it abundantly with all my audiences. It is time for us to realize the importance of touch, movement, human analog sound, music, and curiosity, early on, to assure a bright future for ourselves and our offspring."

—From the Foreword by Carla Hannaford, PhD, author of best-selling books *Smart Moves: Why Learning Is Not All in Your Head,* *The Dominance Factor: How Knowing Your Dominant Eye, Ear, Brain, Hand & Foot Can Improve Your Learning,* and *Playing in the Unified Field: Raising and Becoming Conscious, Creative Human Beings*

Baby Bare

baby bare

A Bottom-Up
Approach to
Growing Strong
Brains and Bodies

Stephanie Johnson, MA, R-DMT, LPC

BABY BARE © copyright 2016 by Stephanie Johnson. All rights reserved. No part of this book may be reproduced in any form whatsoever, by photography or xerography or by any other means, by broadcast or transmission, by translation into any kind of language, nor by recording electronically or otherwise, without permission in writing from the author, except by a reviewer, who may quote brief passages in critical articles or reviews.

ISBN 13: 978-1-63489-038-0

Library of Congress Catalog Number: 2016941590
Printed in the United States of America
Second Printing: 2017
21 20 19 18 17   6 5 4 3 2

Cover and interior design by Ryan Scheife/Mayfly Design
Photographs on pages v, 28, 36, 44-45, 47-49, 55, 62-64, 66-68, 70, 75-78,
    84, 100, and 105 by Kristina Perkins
Photographs on pages vii, 10, 18, 34-43, 47, 50, 54, 56-57, 73, 79, 80, 108,
    and 119 by Meghan Pate
Photograph on page 52 by Laura Cervin
Illustrations by Rachel Beenken

Wise Ink Creative Publishing
837 Glenwood Avenue
Minneapolis, MN 55405
www.wiseinkpub.com

To order, visit babybare.net. Reseller discounts available.

 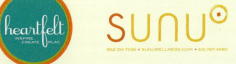

This book is dedicated to children everywhere, whose curiosity must be preserved.

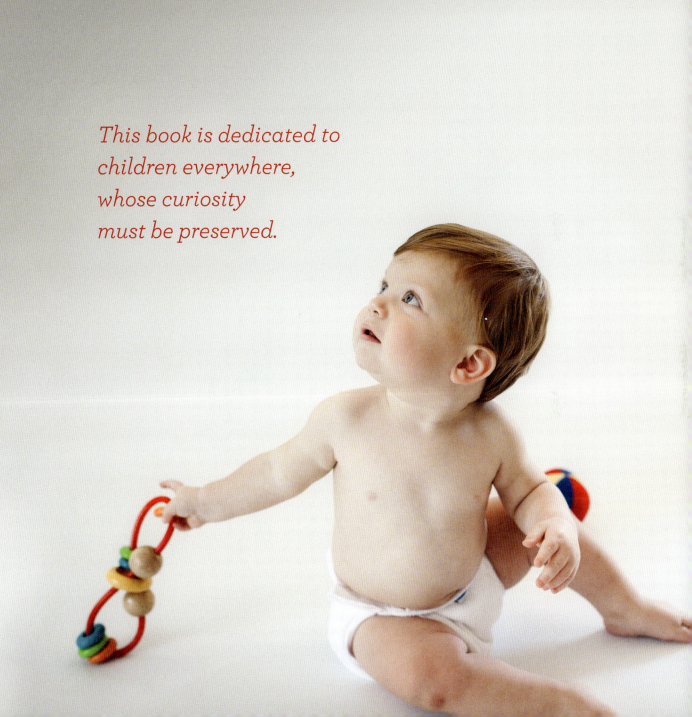

Acknowledgments

I would like to thank those who have taught, inspired, and supported me: Annie Brook, Carla Hannaford, Christine Caldwell, Tom Kanthak, Anne Green Gilbert, Mother Nature, Susan Quigley, Louise Dengerud, Sally Goddard Blythe, Pat Hon, Gideon Wieck, Michael Johnson, Hope Ann McKenzie, Keith Prussing, Joann Parker, Amy Quale, Anitra Budd, Meghan Pate, Kristina Perkins, Graham Johnson, Wendy Johnson, Andre Fischer, Ryan Scheife, Rachel Beenken, Lisa Johnson, Corey Johnson, Brenda Johnson, and all my students and clients who continuously breathe life into this work and fuel my motivation to make an impact.

I'd like to give a very special thanks to Katie Hae Leo, for without her this book quite possibly may not have become a reality. I am forever grateful for your generous spirit and your steadfast belief in me and this work.

And a very, very special thanks to my beloved son, August Fischer, who has brought me the gift of motherhood and all the empathy and wisdom that accompanies it.

Table of Contents

Foreword by Carla Hannaford xiii

Introduction by Stephanie Johnson 1

Chapter 1   The Advantages of Bottom Feeding 11

Chapter 2   Introducing the Triune Brain 19

Chapter 3   Now We're Moving! 29

Chapter 4   Social-Emotional Development 85

Chapter 5   Hemisphere Integration 101

Chapter 6   Our Wonderful Inner Senses 109

Chapter 7   What's Getting in the Way of
Healthy Brain Development? 121

Glossary 135

References and Resources 136

Donor List 137

About the Author 138

Foreword

Seldom does a book grab my interest and extend my understanding of the world in a simple, elegant way that keeps me reading, even with my hectic schedule. This book did just that. It seems parents are looking for answers and often don't trust their innate knowing of how to raise their child. This book shares not only hard-core research but also common sense and instinctual understanding that truly allow parents to enjoy parenting and learn through the eyes of their child.

Learning is the most natural thing we do from before birth on throughout our lives. Babies come into this world as keen observers, mirroring the emotions and beliefs of their parents. We are all compelled to learn new things, but children magnify that learning with their vast curiosity and need to play. Though learning is our nature, a high percentage of school-aged children today are deemed "learning disabled." How can that be?

Stephanie Johnson believes that too often we employ a top-down approach to learning with our children. We drive them to succeed at language, reading, and math early, filling them with facts and information because we believe those signify intelligence. Stephanie, with her bottom-up approach, has elegantly presented current research from developmental experts on what assures whole brain development and lifelong learning success, starting from the very beginning.

From my research and years of sharing how our brains develop, it seems the learning difficulties we see today stem from lack of vestibular development through movement and sound, incompletely integrated early reflexes, and a lack of playful, nurturing human touch and presence from parents and caregivers. In this book, Stephanie supplies us with not only the research but also guidance to assist and optimize our child's learning ability, beginning in utero and continuing throughout the early learning years. She also blesses educators with valuable tools to use in the classroom.

Her examples and visuals make this book a must for every parent, grandparent, and educator. I recommend it highly and plan to share it abundantly with all my audiences. It is time for us to realize the importance of touch, movement, human analog sound, music, and curiosity, early on, to assure a bright future for ourselves and our offspring.

Carla Hannaford, PhD
Author of best-selling books

Smart Moves: Why Learning Is Not All in Your Head,

The Dominance Factor: How Knowing Your Dominant Eye, Ear, Brain, Hand & Foot Can Improve Your Learning, and

Playing in the Unified Field: Raising and Becoming Conscious, Creative Human Beings

Introduction

People often ask me how I came to do this work. The answer is layered. There's the most common layer: I was a teacher who became interested in helping kids individually. But there are also many interesting, less-used layers, and I'd like to share a few with you.

When I look back on my life, I remember instances that were like unconscious whispers guiding me to this work. For example, I myself had difficulty in school; since I was well behaved, none of the adults in my life ever thought anything was wrong. Any signs that school was hard for me were—as with many seemingly bright children—dismissed as proof that I needed to apply myself or work harder. During this time, I remember going to my cement-floored basement after school. I would plug in my mint green cassette player, put on some Prince, and dance. I would choreograph routines and "rehearse" them over and over. I hadn't had any dance training; in fact, I only learned about dance by checking out books about ballet from the library. I would take them home and recreate their pictures with my body. My instinct for health was whispering to me to use movement and my body to help me through those difficult times.

I finally received dance training as a teenager. In my modern dance classes, I began learning the developmental movement patterns that are now the basis of my work. It's funny, because I remember really resisting that part of the classes. I wanted to dance for real, like Coco on *Fame*. I didn't want to roll on the floor like a baby. But even though I hated them, those movements landed deep inside me and became the focal point of my career.

During my college training, I was sure I would become a dancer and choreographer. Dance was my whole life, and I loved every minute of it. It seems strange to look back at that time and imagine choosing anything but dance as a career. I do, however, remember getting a whisper of what was to come during those years.

One day I was taking a break between classes on the steps of the dance building. My whole body was buzzing from the movement and emotion and excitement of the day so far. I loved my life and loved this art form, and I felt as if I could sing it from the mountaintops. Suddenly, a whisper came to me. I remember looking up the road I typically walked home and thinking, *If I left right now and never came back, nobody would be affected at all.* In that moment, I was isolated and lonely, yet I felt so much power and momentum in my body. What a waste of all that energy—I wondered, what was it even for? This feeling lasted for a minute, then I went back to the studios to finish my day.

That moment, in which I felt so much power coursing through me yet having such little positive impact on anyone else, haunted me. Today, I see it as my call to service. Some part of me wanted to serve others, but it hadn't yet found its voice.

Immediately after finishing my undergraduate work in Seattle, I taught dance for the Milwaukee, Wisconsin, public schools. I had no official teacher training, just a BFA in dance. Staff development days were very eye opening for me, for I had no education background at all. I distinctly remember a particularly hard day at a staff development training where I learned that fourth-grade reading scores were often used to predict the number of jail cells that would be needed when those fourth-graders became adults. This knowledge broke my heart, and I wondered what I could do about it as a dance teacher. I began to dabble in educational kinesiology and did some professional development training about the body's role in learning. Throughout the years, I became more interested in advocating for movement in schools because I understood the impact it has on **learning**.

My journey took me from the classroom to a therapeutic setting. There, I work with children who struggle with learning and attention challenges, which are often accompanied by anxiety and/or depression.

The models I use with kids in therapy are based on the development of the nervous system between birth and eighteen months. First, I determine which movement stages were interrupted or incomplete when my clients were babies. We then revisit those stages to reorganize the nervous system and create more joy and ease in the body's ability to perform academically and socially. After working closely with families for years and explaining the work and progress of the children to parents, I hear one thing over and over: "I wish I'd known this when he was a baby!" This is another layer of how I came to this work. Developmental movement therapy can be used to great effect with school-aged children. But what if new parents understood the importance of completing each movement stage with their newborns?

> "I wish I'd known this when he was a baby!"

I became committed to offering a proactive approach, one that builds strong brains and bodies from the first day of a child's life. We know what children need to develop optimally—why wait until there's a problem at school? I developed movement classes for new parents and taught them to both parents and educators around Minneapolis. As I did, I began to realize people were interested in learning more. Today, I spend half my time educating new families and half doing therapy with older children and adults.

School-Aged Children

School-aged children come to see me with a wide range of symptoms that can impede them from sharing their gifts with the world. Some have more traditional mental health symptoms, others struggle academically, and still others fall into the category of "we can't put our finger on it, but we know he needs support." Their families typically come because they're looking for another perspective than the ones other well-meaning professionals involved in the child's development are offering. The way I work—uncovering the underlying origin of symptoms rather than providing a series of coping mechanisms or accommodations—resonates with many parents. Others are drawn to the movement aspect of the work. Whatever brings them in, they all want to support their child in a noninvasive way. Together, we focus on reorganizing the nervous system and emphasizing that there is nothing wrong with their child; things just need to be adjusted a bit.

You see, when children arrive at school, they're expected to have what I call "invisible mechanics of learning." These include the ability to focus on a task, sit still in a chair, exhibit awareness of their body in space, organize their desks as well as their thoughts, regulate emotions, and so on. These skills are necessary for optimal school achievement; however, in many schools, little is done to develop these skills; your child is expected to arrive with them in place.

For the most part, these invisible mechanics of learning are hardwired into the nervous system during the first eighteen months of life. They are strengthened over the years and become more refined as children mature, but the birth of the learning body and brain starts before the child is born. I like to think of the body as being in service to the brain. For example, a child takes a field trip to the zoo and is very excited about the snake he saw slithering and slinking in its habitat. When he gets back to the classroom, the teacher asks the children to write a poem and draw a picture of their favorite animal. His brain has a lot of ideas and imagery to express, but what does the expressing? What gets those ideas out of his head and into the world? The answer: his body. The body is often taken for granted, but think of all it does: his bottom half must stabilize so his top half can move; one hand has to stabilize so the other can move; his hand has to move and act like a mouthpiece for his brain in order for him to get his ideas across. In other words, his body is in service to his brain.

> I like to think of the body as being in service to the brain.

In an ideal situation, all these invisible mechanics are in place so the child can freely and joyfully articulate the images and thoughts he has about that slinking snake. My clients, though very bright and filled with ideas, cannot count on their bodies to act as mouthpieces for their brains. Those invisible mechanics are not in place, making it difficult for them to express themselves. Since this type of child development is not part of teacher training, it's common for well-meaning teachers to tell bright children whose bodies do not support their brains that they simply need to try harder or apply themselves. The reality is, these children are often working harder than their peers.

School readiness begins before we are born. We don't rush it; it develops naturally in the right environment. But preparing the body for learning is a large piece of child development that is being overlooked while we spend so much money and energy on finding the perfect, magical teaching tools, pushing early academics, and often pointing fingers at teachers when we don't get the desired results. The truth is, preparing children from the ground up can go a long way to improving the academic lives of our youth.

Infants

When babies come to me for their Baby Bare Milestone Checkups, I spend most of the time educating parents on the value of each movement stage as well as assessing the baby's development. There are early indicators of whether the baby will experience difficulty with any of the movement stages, and it is typically easier to provide gentle treatment and play ideas to facilitate completion of each stage than it is to revisit missed stages later on as a school-aged child.

I work with new families who want to learn about movement and brain development. As you can imagine, it's tricky to get a parent to seek out a professional unless there's a concern. In our culture, we have a relationship to wellness that keeps us waiting until we see a problem. Even when we do, we often ignore it and hope the issue will resolve itself. It's only when the problem grows too big to ignore that we find a professional. I help parents get in front of any concerns by learning about the pieces of optimal development and how simple they are to implement.

I am so passionate about empowering parents with this information that for the first few years of my work I actually offered free visits to families with newborns. It continues to be a huge effort to get families to see the value of proactive education. I'm often faced with people who say things like, "My niece went straight from rolling to walking, and she's just fine." My response is, "Great, I'm so glad your niece is doing well! However, I have a practice full of clients who aren't doing so well, and the nation is full of children in the same position." It certainly is possible to skip stages during infancy and still be "fine," but at what cost? Also, while humans are equipped with immense powers of compensation when our systems don't work efficiently, compensating can be very hard on the nervous system. The point is this: There is no risk in taking steps early on to ensure optimal development, so why not do it? I'm reminded of Frederick Douglass's famous quote: "It's easier to raise strong children than to mend broken men." We can't guarantee that if your child skips crawling, she will have difficulty reading, but why take the risk?

How to Use This Book

Whether you're reading this book while pregnant or have a wiggly seven-month-old in your arms, let me first congratulate you on this exciting new journey of parenting! This book introduces theories and concepts in a way that's easy to digest and apply to your baby. (If you're looking to dive more deeply into brain development, check out the reference and resources section at the end of the book!)

Those of you who are pregnant may feel as if you want to read everything you can get your hands on. You may also be feeling an urge to nest and get your home ready for the baby. You may enjoy reading this book cover to cover to get your fill of concepts and theory, as well as yummy baby photos!

If you came across this book after delivery, you may find yourself a bit sleep deprived and not feeling up to a cover-to-cover reading commitment. For you, I say flip to the part of the book that describes the stage your baby is in. You will find photos of what your baby is doing during that stage, easy-to-use tips for promoting stage-appropriate development, and information on why the stage is important later in her life. If you feel like getting back to the theory chapters later, that's great. This book was designed to help exhausted and overwhelmed new parents, so flipping through may be the way to go.

The sequence of movements and experiencing them all is more important than the age at which the child is able to perform the movement. The ages associated with each stage are general and each baby will develop at his own pace. A baby who has completed all the stages and walks at fifteen months has a great foundation for optimal physical, cognitive, and emotional development. There is no value in baby skipping stages and walking at nine months. As you read this book, you will begin to understand the value of

> The sequence of movements and experiencing them all is more important than the age at which the child is able to perform the movement.

each stage and see how walking early does not mean a baby is advanced and smarter than later walkers. There is no "testing out" of developmental stages; they each offer a unique and crucial opportunity for development that can only be attained by experiencing them fully.

Wherever you are in your parenting journey, I encourage you to reflect inward for as many minutes as you read this or any other book. I always tell the parents I work with, "If you read a parenting book for thirty minutes, do whatever brings you closer to your internal source of knowing and wisdom—taking a bath, meditating, praying, taking a walk, going for a swim, practicing yoga—for thirty minutes as well." We must balance what is outside with what is inside. This practice will serve you throughout your parenting journey. When it comes right down to it, your inner wisdom in relationship to your child trumps anything experts say (and "experts" includes well-intentioned grandparents!). I might know a lot about babies and movement, your parents may have raised five children, and your pediatrician may know a lot about vaccinations, but you are intimately connected to the child in your arms or belly. That bond is what will guide you. If you don't read another page of this book, please know that you already have everything you need to care for your baby.

This book gently invites you to learn about those little wiggly bundles and all they are designed to do. The suggestions in these pages are just that: suggestions. Try what resonates with you at any given time. This book is for you, dear new mama and papa. Congratulations—you are part of the universal network of parents. Please know that though you will feel isolated at times, we are all out here trying to do the best we can for our children. Welcome!

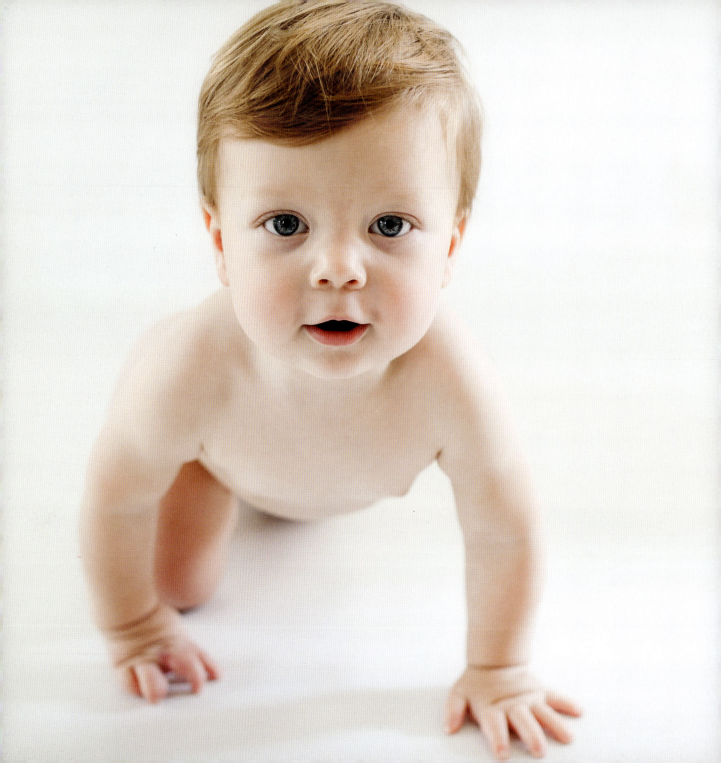

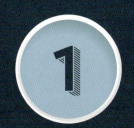

The Advantages of Bottom Feeding

When I say "bottom feeder," most people think of something negative. But when it comes to child development, bottom feeding is actually ideal. Modern-day neuroscience has proven this, and many wise grandmothers have always known it. But what do I mean by "bottom feeding"? In this chapter, I'll explain more as we look at two approaches to developing the human brain—top down and bottom up.

The Top-Down Approach

If you're like me, you probably grew up with the idea that children are empty containers, ready for adults to fill with information and knowledge. In the top-down approach, a teacher, parent, or other well-meaning adult fills the child with facts and information. Letters of the alphabet, numbers, geography, math—all the things we adults associate with intelligence. Sometimes we ask the child to recite these things back to us, and sometimes we even like to have them recite to family or friends. We've all experienced that four-year-old who can count to fifty or name the capital of Wyoming as his proud parents look on.

Who can blame the parent? Adults measure intelligence by our command of facts and information and our ability to communicate them. We associate strong verbal skills with a powerful brain. We know that acquiring language is good and that reading is good, therefore reading early must be *extra* good. So we encourage our children to read as early as possible, sometimes even sitting them in front of videos that promise to give them an edge over their peers. And when we see a four-year-old who can mimic facts and information back at us, we naturally say to ourselves, "What a smart child!" This child has been reared using the top-down approach. His brain has been nurtured without appreciation for his body's role in laying the foundation for all that knowledge.

What will happen to that child five years down the road? This bright, vibrant child who loves learning and whose brain is filled with so much sophisticated knowledge will go to school. He will need to hold a pencil or pen and write. He will need to move his eyes from left to right across a page, keeping track of where he is. He will need to sit still in his chair for long stretches of time while using his upper body to perform different tasks. All of this work requires a body with properly developed mechanics. When mechanics are developed, it frees up higher brain functions for higher learning. But if a child's brain has not been appropriately primed in this way, he will struggle and possibly start to fall behind. And if his physical ability to learn continues to impede his academic progress, he may eventually believe school is not for him. This is why the bottom-up approach is so important. It understands that successful learning must be, first and foremost, grounded in the body. Ideally, the body serves as a tool of expression for what the brain is learning. When we only focus on filling the brain with facts, we are missing a big part of what makes us whole, expressive beings.

The Bottom-Up Approach

As a parent, educator, and therapist, I know that in order for a child to achieve optimum learning, she must first possess the necessary body mechanics to acquire that learning. In other words, the human body is essential to education. This may sound counterintuitive. We've been told for many years that the brain is essential to education. But the brain and body are connected, and our bodies actually feed our brains. During the earliest months and years of life, the movements of babies' bodies create blueprints in their brains for skills they will need in the future. These early months are absolutely crucial for your baby.

The bottom-up approach to child development understands that physical movement early in life builds parts of the brain that children will need later. It asks, "How can we get children's bodies ready so they are able to receive, absorb, and express knowledge later on?" For example, one of the mechanisms a body needs to read proficiently at grade level is horizontal

> "How can we get children's bodies
> ready so they are able to receive, absorb,
> and express knowledge later on?"

eye tracking, or scanning from left to right (in English and other Western languages). The body's ability to physically sit still and scan from left to right across a page is developed during that window of birth to eighteen months. The primitive movements a baby makes will create the blueprint in her lower brain for future reading. If this blueprint has been created and nurtured in her brain as a baby, when she begins to read, her eye tracking will be automatic. She won't have to worry about the mechanics and can instead concentrate on decoding symbols, interpreting content, and other skills associated with the higher brain.

But, if she skips the body mechanics and goes directly to higher order thinking as in the top-down approach, then chances are this child will struggle later in school, no matter how much information she has acquired.

About This Book

Baby Bare takes the bottom-up approach to child development. It views bodily movement as a crucial tool for building a child's brain and looks at ways we adults both help and hinder this growth.

Imagine two oak trees in a forest. One grows very fast, so fast that once it reaches maturity,

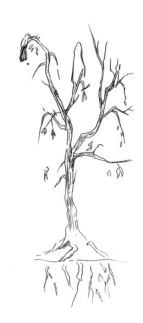

This tree grew so fast that it didn't have time to grow deep roots and strong branches; that takes time, just like growing strong brains and bodies. There is no rush to walking—slow down and enjoy the journey.

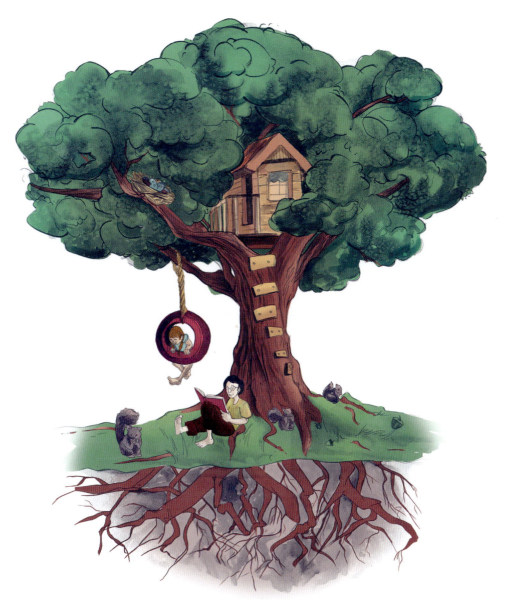

Just like a slowly growing oak tree whose roots grow deep and branches grow strong, a child who is allowed the time and space to grow slow and steady from the bottom up will have so much to offer the world.

it remains thin and rather flimsy. It cannot withstand wind or rain storms, and it blows this way and that in harsh weather. It has very little to offer—no shade, no acorns, no shelter, and no strong branches for climbing. The other oak tree has grown slowly and deliberately. Its roots reach deep into the earth, enabling it to withstand a great deal. Through wind and storms, it bends and adapts itself, because it has such a firm grounding. It has much to offer—lots of shade and acorns, shelter for passersby, and strong branches for children to climb.

We want our children to become strong yet flexible, like the second oak tree. This book will teach you some ways to help your baby grow in this way.

Summary

- Childhood is not a race; there is value to allowing children to grow slowly.
- Our culture is focused on a top-down approach to child development that does not recognize the body's important role in brain development.
- The bottom-up approach to child development honors the body's role in brain development. This approach encourages optimal development through movement in preparation for academic pursuits rather than pushing early academic learning.

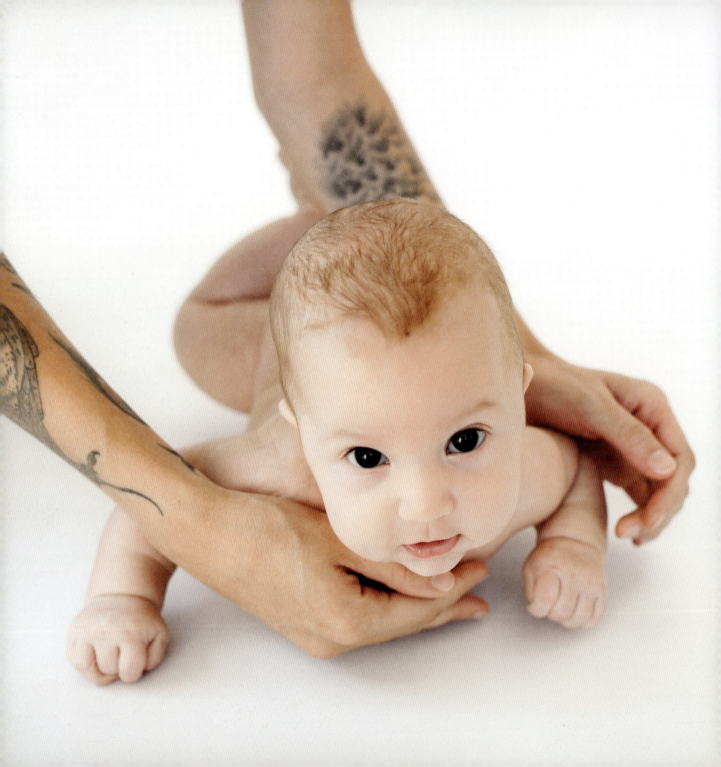

2

Introducing the Triune Brain

I will never forget the first time I looked at my beautiful baby boy August right after he was born. Like you, I knew at that moment I would do anything to ensure that this precious being could develop into his best possible self. As someone trained in early childhood neurological development, I also knew that even as an infant, August's brain and body were already equipped with everything they needed to grow. And as his mother, one of my primary jobs was simply to allow this growth to happen.

The Triune Brain

> "Our higher cognitive processes are grounded in bodily experience, such that the sensory and motor neural circuits do not just feed into cognition, they *are* cognition."
>
> —Arthur Glenberg,
> *Embodiment as a Unifying Perspective for Psychology*

Scientists today have many different ways of explaining the human brain, with lots of specific and technical names for its various parts and functions. While the brain works as a whole, we can still study its parts to better understand the bottom-up approach.

For our purposes, we are going to use something called the triune brain theory (Maclean, 1968). Basically, this means we will focus on three areas of the brain (the "tri" in triune) as we consider childhood development. These areas are the hindbrain (pronounced as in "behind"), the midbrain, and the neocortex. Our body position plays a role in what area of the brain we utilize. When we are on the floor, we access the hindbrain; when we are mid-level as in creeping on all fours, we best access the midbrain; and when we are fully upright, we have the best access to the cortex. To help us remember the roles of the hindbrain, midbrain, and neocortex, it is sometimes helpful to use these images: alligator for hindbrain, elephant for midbrain, and a sturdy, upright adult for the neocortex.

The Hindbrain

A mature adult brain works as an integrated whole, but there are windows of development that will help us further appreciate the bottom-up approach. The optimal window for hindbrain development is from birth to eighteen months, while the cortex continues to grow until early adulthood. The long window of cortex development, as compared to the relatively short window for hindbrain development, invites us to slow down and let the hindbrain have its time. There is no need to rush past this crucial hindbrain development time to get to reading and calculating.

The hindbrain sits at the top of the spine and regulates all the things we don't need to spend time consciously thinking about, such as heart function, lung function, digestion, and temperature. It controls our responses to stimuli, including our "fight-or-flight" mechanism and all reflexes, as well as blinking, swallowing, and breathing. Think of it as the seat of everything automatic, or the "bottom" of the brain.

The alligator reminds us of the importance of activities that happen on the floor. Our progress-oriented adult brains may tend to believe that movement on the floor, like crawling, is less important than upright movement like walking. But, in the bottom-up approach, we know all the work babies do on the floor is absolutely essential for building powerful brains. In order for your

> the work babies do on the floor is absolutely essential for building powerful brains

baby to reach her full potential, movement on the floor must receive its due time and space because the floor is where the hindbrain is best developed.

Remember, the hindbrain regulates automatic functions; therefore, skills acquired on the floor become regulated by the hindbrain and are automatic for life. For example: When your baby is happily spending time on the floor on her tummy, there will come a time when she sees something interesting that she wants to reach for, grab, and no doubt bring to her mouth for a closer "look." To do that, she will need to lean into one arm, allowing the other arm to do the reaching, grabbing, and bringing to the mouth. Since they were done on the floor, that sequence of movements will now be an automatic one that she can rely on forever. Her body has made the act of keeping one arm grounded while the other moves routine; one arm can do something different than the other. Eating, writing, playing the violin, painting, throwing a ball—all depend on the unconscious ability to do something different with each arm. This is only one example of how the hindbrain, if properly developed, serves the higher parts of the brain for life. It's the bottom-up approach: the bottom feeds the upper! When you know that the hindbrain has the shortest window for optimal development, you can begin to see the importance of focusing on its development first.

The Midbrain

The midbrain, also known as the limbic system, is made up of complex, specialized parts that regulate emotions, memory, and learning. Think of it as the gateway from the hindbrain to the cortex as it connects parts of the brain that deal with high and low functions.

We have all seen a toddler experience surges of emotion, often with no regard for the setting or impact on himself or others. These demonstrations of unbridled emotion are a sign that the limbic system is developing, but since the neocortex is still so underdeveloped, the child is unable to regulate his big emotions on his own and needs a caring adult to assist. Although parts of the limbic system like the amygdala are fully developed in utero, other parts are still developing when your baby is a toddler; the hippocampus, for example, is thought to be fully developed between the ages of three and five.

The amygdala and hippocampus are both implicated in memory, but each has a different role. The amygdala holds the emotional part of the memory, what we feel about an experience. The hippocampus is host to our declarative memory, which is the story line of the experience. People often say we don't have our first memories until we are about five; what that really means is that while we may not have words for an incident until we are five, we certainly have memories of how experiences made us feel.

Since the amygdala is fully formed in utero, we have plenty of feeling memories. This is why, as parents, it is of the utmost importance to give our babies a sense of love, warmth, and protection. What babies feel about every experience they have is stored and used later to recognize and prepare for future experiences.

Moving freely and physically interacting with the three-dimensional world with a sense of love and protection primes young minds to feel safe when exploring their world in increasingly complex ways. As your baby becomes more mobile and explorative, you can support optimal midbrain development by offering a balance of freedom and protection. Babies will begin by crawling away a bit, then look back and see Mom or Dad is still there. This interplay between limbic development and independence in the physical form is a dance you will enjoy with your older baby and into the toddler years. Providing a safe environment for baby will be key in developing a perception of safety in the world. We will learn more about how to do this in later chapters.

The midbrain has a longer window of development than the hindbrain and contributes to emotional development and memory. We often pair midbrain development with more independent mobilizing on all fours, creeping, cruising, and toddling. You can read more about these movement stages in chapter 3.

The Neocortex

The neocortex, also known as the frontal cortex or sometimes just the cortex, gives us much of what makes us uniquely human. Creativity, foresight, hindsight, the ability to reflect on experience, imagination, fantasy, and the ability to decode symbols all reside here. It sits like a swim cap on top of our head and is full of beautiful folds and wrinkles. The cortex is divided into two hemispheres commonly referred to as the right and left brain. Each hemisphere has specialized areas of strength and throughout life we rely of the hemispheres communicating with each other. We call this communication between right and left sides "hemisphere integration." We will talk more about the process of hemisphere integration in chapter 5. Although it is the neocortex that is responsible for higher-order thinking, the lower parts of the brain need a solid foundation for the neocortex to blossom and express its remarkable capacity. In this book, you will often hear me say that the low brain, when allowed to develop optimally, will be in service of the cortex for our whole lives. What I mean by that is that the tools of expression that allow us to both take in and share sophisticated ideas and thoughts rely heavily in our ability to use our bodies to communicate with speech, gesture, written language, music, etc. This part of the brain has the longest window of development, with some research stating it is not developed fully until early adulthood.

A bottom-up approach to child development values the long-term journey of the neocortex and emphasizes the strong development of the hind- and midbrain first, rather than rush children to use the neocortex before developing a strong foundation. There is no rush; the cortex needs a sturdy platform to stand on, and this book will help you understand how to ensure your child's hindbrain is getting just what it needs to be that sturdy foundation of learning.

Our upright vertical posture is associated with the neocortex. When we are upright we are best able to access the cortex. Think of how the astronauts train for their missions to space where their vertical body position is

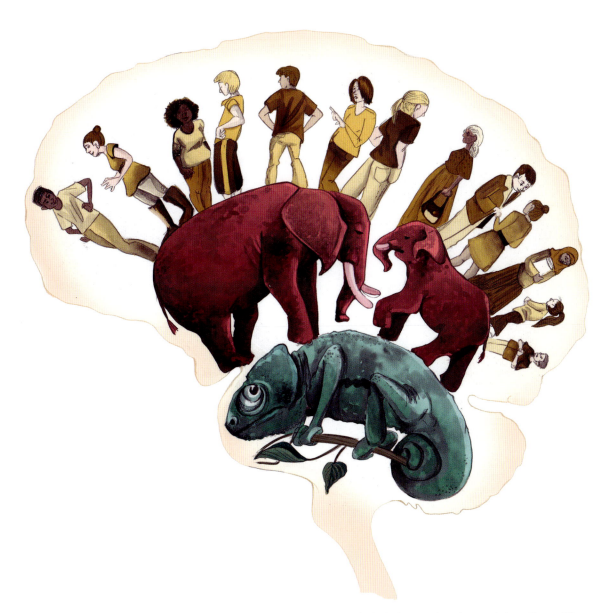

The lower parts of the brain have a shorter window of optimal development, while the higher parts have longer windows. Plenty of floor time during infancy is crucial for optimal hindbrain development and will ensure that the hindbrain can be in lifelong service to the cortex.

Introducing the Triune Brain

compromised. They practice in simulators that have their body floating in all different planes. It is very hard to access the higher parts of the brain when you are upside down or even lying down. Remember our reptile: the low brain is in use when we are lying down, therefore special training is needed to do tasks that require the cortex while the body is upside down, as in space exploration. Now think about how a baby spends most of its time these days: 75 percent of a baby's day is spent in a container that props her up in the vertical position. This means the cortex is being prematurely developed while precious time on the floor developing the hindbrain is being lost. This contributes to the negative aspects of the top-down approach. Early cortex development creates very thoughtful, verbal young children whose bodies will not be able to support their highly developed cortex throughout life. Throughout this book you will learn ways to ensure your baby is getting enough time on the floor and less time in the containing devices.

The Triune Brain and the Bottom-Up Approach

The development of each of the three parts of the brain is cyclical and ongoing. However, for the purposes of our bottom-up approach, we will think of the hindbrain as having the shortest window for optimal development, followed by the midbrain, then the neocortex having the longest development window, extending into young adulthood. This sequence lets us consider the chain of events needed for the healthy development of each part. Think of infant brain development as a stairway. To reach the next level, we must ensure the level we are on has the proper foundation.

The first months and years of your baby's life are vitally important. In that precious time, his brain is developing all the skills he will need to use at school, work, and play. I cannot overstate how crucial the body is to this work. Remember, in our bottom-up approach, the body feeds the brain. Your infant's brain learns through his body. He does not yet have the complex mechanisms that adults have to take in and process intellectual information. The healthiest, most effective way to build your child's brain is by allowing him to move in a safe, loving environment.

Summary

- While there are many ways to divide and examine the brain, we are concerned with the triune brain theory, which considers the brain in three sections: hindbrain, midbrain, and neocortex.
- We are especially concerned with the hindbrain since it is foundational to brain development and all future growth and has a small window of optimal development—conception to approximately eighteen months.
- Remember, a well-developed hindbrain will serve your child for life. All future ideas and cognitive pursuits will be best expressed by old movement patterns tucked away in the hindbrain.
- A sense of safety and freedom of movement are key to optimal hindbrain development.
- In this book, we will explore many different ways for you to help your child grow his brain, focusing on natural movements as the basis.

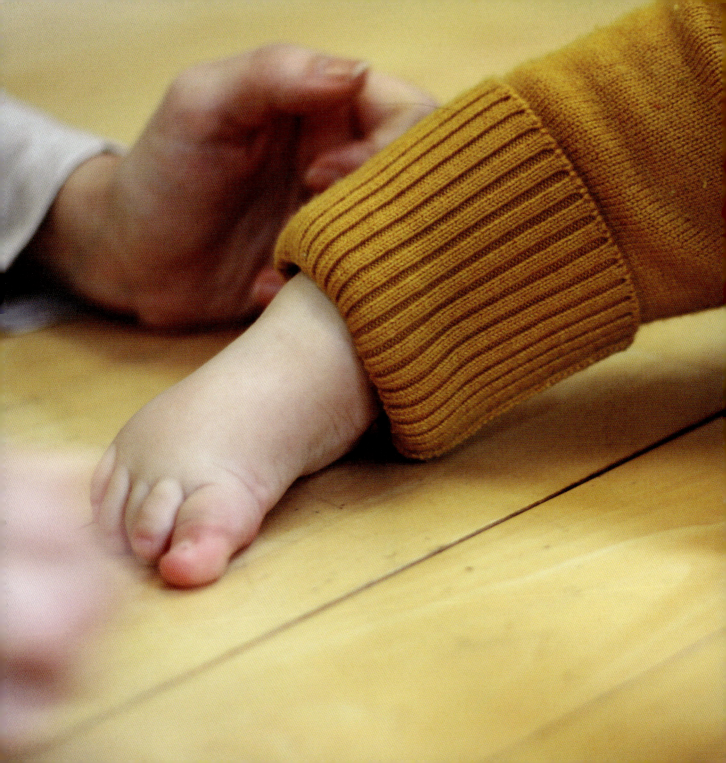

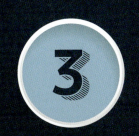

Now We're Moving!

In the bottom-up approach to child development, we know a baby develops her brain through her body. Free movement is a key component to growing a strong hindbrain, which will in turn feed her cortex and prepare her for future learning. When we say "learning," it is important to note the expression and demonstration of the learning is also important. In my practice, I see many bright students who are definitely learning, but they struggle with the output of that learning. Homework, writing, drawing, organization—are all problematic because early on in their development, the cortex was overly stimulated before the hindbrain had time to develop. As a result, they have all the right ideas and answers and language skills, but their bodies have not been prepared to express them, leading them to fall behind in school and often putting their self-esteem and confidence at risk.

Remember that your baby has a window from conception to eighteen months for developing her hindbrain optimally. As the hindbrain develops, it stimulates the higher parts of the brain. In this chapter we will look at the different stages of your baby's growth as they would occur in an optimal setting. This includes what you will likely see in each stage, how it relates to later learning, and how best to make sure your baby moves freely through the development process.

Flexion and Extension

Picture a sunflower and how it opens and closes according to its natural rhythms. In the first weeks of your baby's life, her body is like this sunflower. Her first movements will be to open to the world and close back in—open, close, open, close. When her body folds in, she is in **flexion**; when her body stretches out, she is in **extension**.

Flexion and extension are the most basic components of all movement. The flexor muscles are located along the front of the body. Flexion occurs when you fold your joints; sitting at your desk typing, you are mostly using

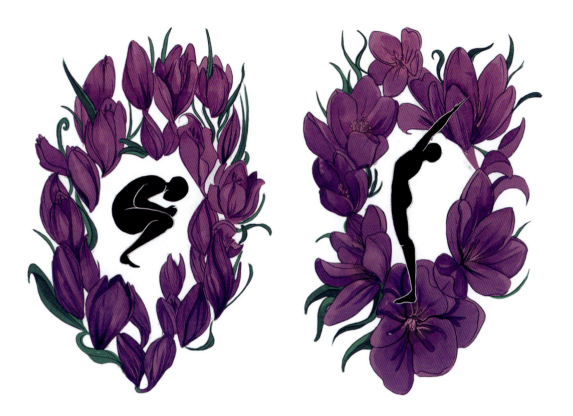

The basic alphabet of all movement is flexion and extension. This natural opening and closing starts first as a whole-body movement and will become more complex in the next few months. The balance between flexion and extension is crucial for optimal development.

flexion. Extension occurs when you straighten your joints. If you reach across a table to grab a drink, your arm is in extension. When you bring the glass to your mouth, you fold into flexion. All movement is a complex orchestration of these two basic components.

Your baby's first movements involve the whole body. When she arches, the extensor muscles on her back activate, and all six of her limbs extend away from her center. (We count the limbs as two arms, two legs, one head, and one tail.) When your baby flexes, those limbs contract, and her whole body folds into itself. These movements are involuntary at first, then become more purposeful over time.

As your baby grows, she'll start to move certain parts of her body separately, opening and folding them like an origami crane or those little folded paper notes we used to pass in school. She will discover how to move her head and tail, then her upper and lower body, then her left and right side, and so on. It's thrilling for parents to witness their children discovering parts of their bodies on their own. With that in mind, let's look at some beautiful babies and the different stages of early movement—get ready for an exciting and fun journey!

Primitive Reflexes

How does baby know about these movements? Baby has a series of primitive reflexes that are innate and scheduled to emerge during the early months. Primitive reflexes are different than lifelong reflexes, such as those that keep us safe from leaving our finger on a hot kettle for too long. That type of reflex causes us to pull the finger away quickly, and we rely on these lifelong reflexes into adulthood. Primitive reflexes have a much different role—they are designed to help babies during the birth process and orient them to their new environment after birth. Think of them as the blueprint of movement. Each primitive reflex has a specific role in your baby's movement journey. The lifecycle of a primitive reflex is as such: one reflex emerges, does its job, and then integrates into the hindbrain so that more sophisticated and purposeful movement can build off of it. For example, there is a primitive reflex that tells baby to lift his head when he is on his tummy on the floor. After that reflex has done its job of whispering to baby to lift his head and baby has practiced that head lifting for a period of time, the reflex integrates or tucks away and makes possible the purposeful movement of baby turning his head to watch the dog run by or turning toward Dad's voice. In addition to allowing for fancier, voluntary movement, the integration of one reflex can also act as a trigger for the next primitive reflex to emerge. This series of primitive reflexes creates the foundation for each movement your baby will make and is innate.

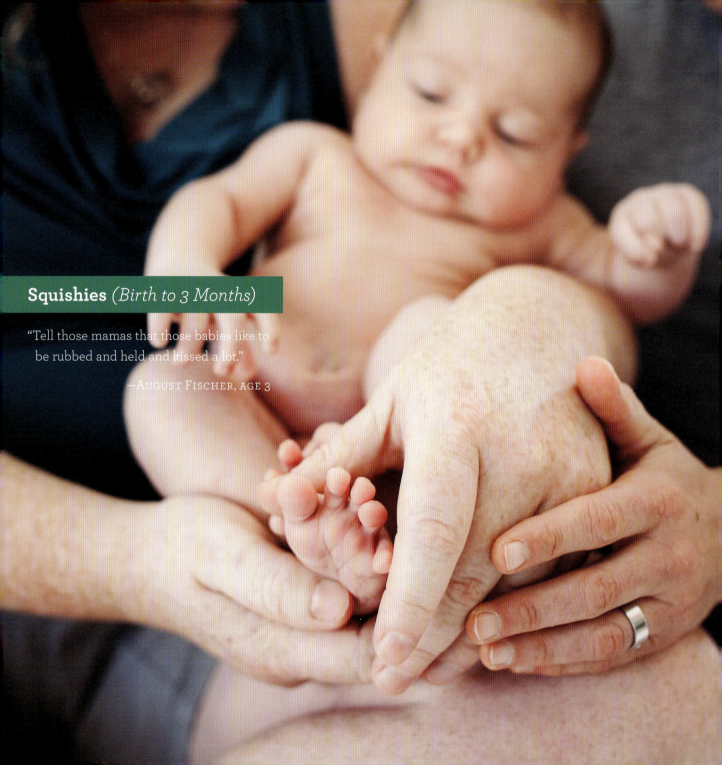

Squishies *(Birth to 3 Months)*

"Tell those mamas that those babies like to be rubbed and held and kissed a lot."

—August Fischer, age 3

Think of the first three months of your baby's life as the fourth trimester. Your baby's system is very immature and fragile and above all needs closeness and love to thrive. Cherish this invitation to slow down and keep it simple. This is the time for gaining flexion and extension for every other stage baby will experience. Baby develops balance between flexion and extension during these first months; her head becomes stable in the center of her body, and her hands and feet fold in toward the center of her body. During this stage, she gains stabilization along three axes—transverse, horizontal, and vertical.

When baby is born she has very little strength. When placed on her back she will first be folded from the position of her body in utero, but will eventually allow her limbs to open in a floppy manner out to the side. Bringing arms, legs, and head to the center of the body in the supine position is baby's first job. She is developing her flexion strength. When baby's head and body are stabilized, she can begin to visually track objects without moving her head.

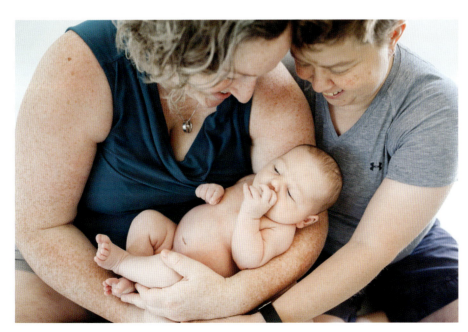

Closeness trumps everything else at this stage; keep baby close.

Now We're Moving!

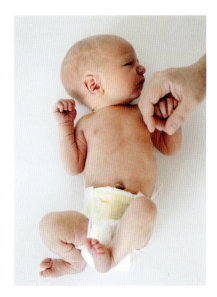 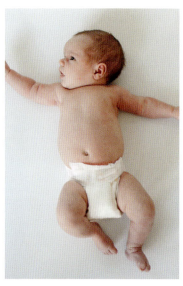 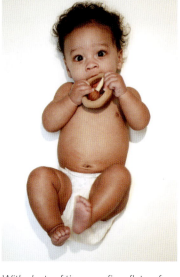

Gryffin is still curled up tight shortly after delivery. Proximity is the most important thing for him now.

Linus begins to relax and unfold, but still very little extension or flexion strength.

With plenty of time on a firm, flat surface, Nelson has developed flexion strength, his head is centered, and his arms and legs are pulled into the center of his body; he is establishing his midline. Once his head is stable in the center, he can use his eyes to start tracking objects. This independent eye tracking is crucial for reading words and music on the page when he's older.

We call this independent eye tracking. Independent eye tracking is crucial for a number of activities later in life, including reading words and music and watching moving objects. Placing baby on her back on a firm, flat surface is the best way to encourage this front flexion.

Short, frequent durations of time on her tummy are also important at this stage. Baby may enjoy tummy time most when she's placed on your stomach or when you're down on the floor with her. Place baby on her tummy without moving her arms forward—she will learn to do this on her own. If you do it for her, it may interrupt the balance between flexion and extension.

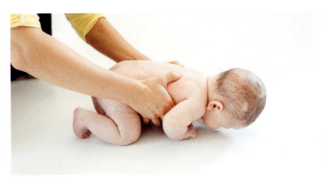

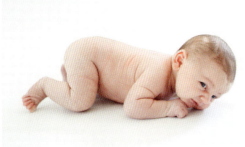

Gus is being placed on his tummy. Just as he is, he will learn to move his own arms and that will help him build flexion and extension strength.

What You Will See in the Squishy Stage

- Lifting head
- Turning head from side to side once strong in center
- Gazing at faces
- Responding to facial expressions. Baby may copy your mouth and tongue movements.
- Waving arms and kicking legs
- Putting hands in mouth
- Turning head toward a sound
- Visually tracking objects
- Bringing hands together while on back
- Bringing feet together while on back
- Head stabilizing at midline (head stabilizing on neck)
- Watching hands
- Purposeful grasping
- Touching your face and hair with both hands
- Beginning to laugh or vocalize more
- Beginning to have weight on hands while on tummy

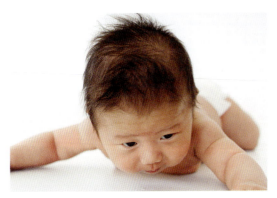

Yuto attempting to lift his head for the first time!

Now We're Moving!

Squishies

Cameron and Daddy getting a little face time!

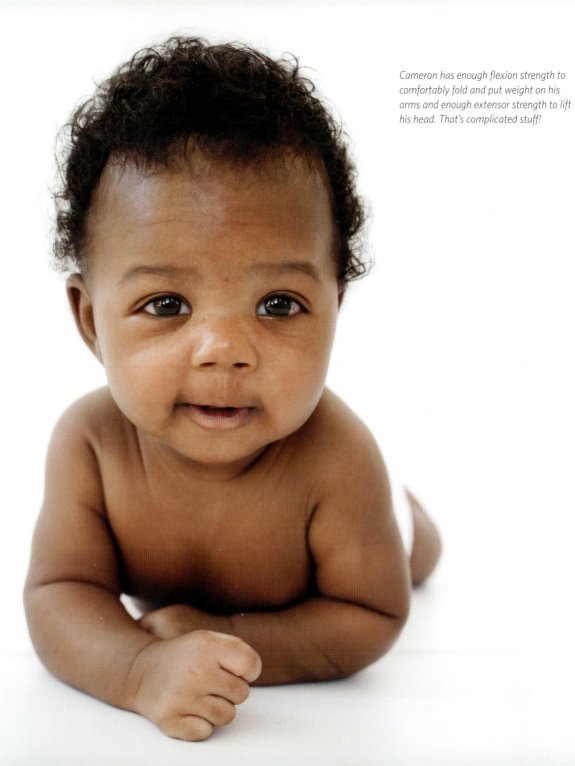

Cameron has enough flexion strength to comfortably fold and put weight on his arms and enough extensor strength to lift his head. That's complicated stuff!

Squishies

Squishies

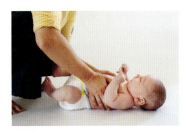

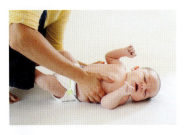

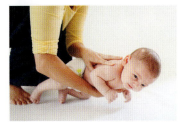

Gus is being rolled over to the side before being picked up. This will help keep his limbs in flexion during transition and will help him feel safe and supported.

Ways to Support Baby's Squishy Stage

- Roll baby to the side before picking her up
- Talk and sing to baby
- Let baby feel your face and pull your hair
- Let baby feel your hands and put them in her mouth
- Let baby experience his own voice, and copy those sounds with your own
- Provide plenty of naked free time; diapers can restrict leg and hip movement. The best time for naked play is after baby has been changed, when you have a little time before the next soiled diaper. If you're concerned about getting the floor dirty, use a towel or "potty pad," which can be found at pet stores.
- Lift baby's limbs one at a time and apply deep, gentle pressure on the joints
- If baby is happy, let her lie there
- Hold and gently rock baby
- Feed baby on both sides
- Spend most time with baby on back with frequent, short durations on the tummy

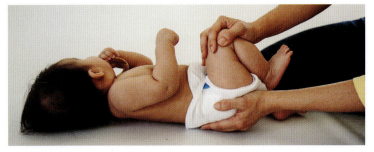

Lift baby's joints one at a time and apply deep, gentle pressure on the joints. This is especially helpful for babies who may have difficulty folding into the center. Babies that seem to have stiff legs and arms will have trouble with the upcoming movement stages, and this deep pressure can really help balance the flexion and extension.

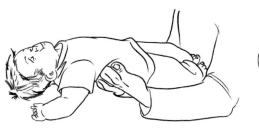 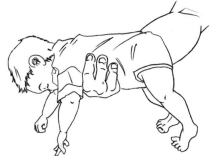

The way we typically pick up infants does not support the calm, inward flexion that is needed to help very young infants feel safe.

This baby's body is favoring extension. Deep compression to the joints, as well as plenty of time on the back, will help soften the extension and invite more flexion so that baby can move with ease through the upcoming movement stages.

What to Avoid in the Squishy Stage

- Don't offer toys to baby until she can bring her hands together at the center, generally around three months. Her hands will be her first toys.
- Don't stand baby on her feet or let her jump
- Don't pull baby up by her hands into a sitting position
- Don't place baby in a device that props her up or puts her body at an incline
- Never leave baby in a car seat when you're not in the car. Keep a baby wrap or carrier handy for transporting baby.
- When carrying baby in a front pack, don't place her facing forward. Not only can forward placement compromise the development of the hip sockets, but meeting all that sensory input from the world without your protection can also be scary for baby.

Squishies

- Don't encourage or try to force baby to accelerate through stages to get to the next one
- Protect baby from media screens and/or television

Tips for Adults

- Sleep when baby sleeps
- Take warm baths
- Drink plenty of water
- Eat frequent, small meals high in healthy fats and proteins
- Take long, deep breaths
- Engage in gentle movement every day
- Keep loved ones near when possible and use your support system

Shayan is lucky to have so much love and support, this will help mom transition to motherhood and help Shayan's brain grow!

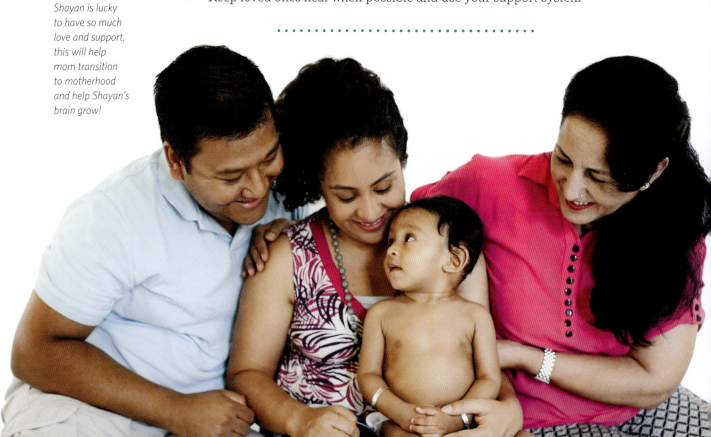

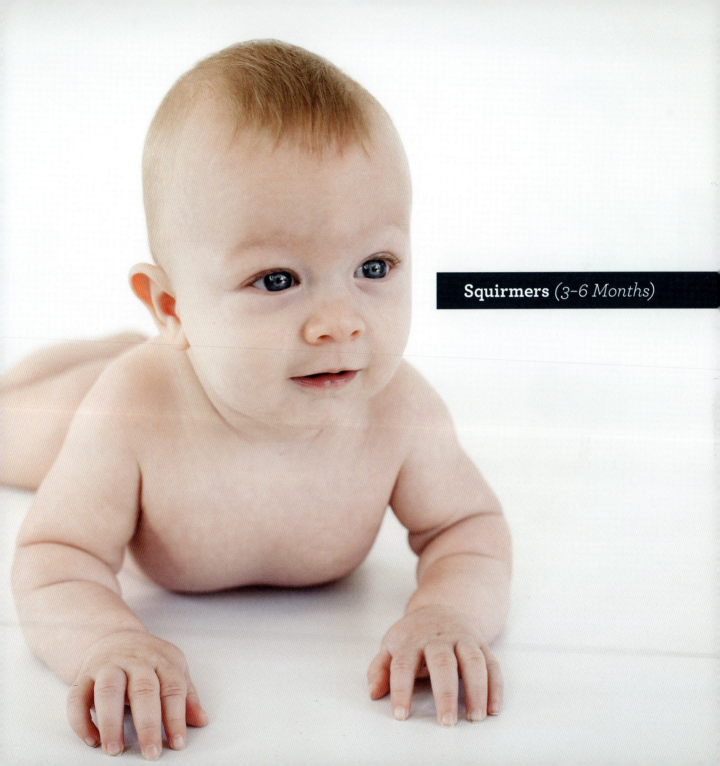

Squirmers

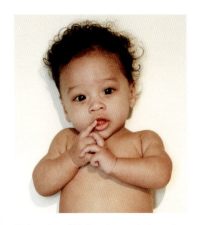

Nelson found his hands, now he's ready for a toy! There is no need to offer your baby a toy before his hands meet in the middle and he explores his hands with his mouth.

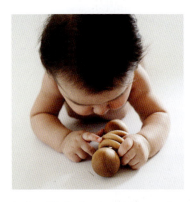

Luciana lifts her head and folds arms in to explore a toy with two hands. To do this, she is grounding through her lower body and establishing her center. Both of these things will help her sit and focus when the time comes.

Squirmers are awake to the world around them, and they are starting to use their bodies to explore it. You will see their attention focus outward as they get to know their surroundings and draw back for periods of recuperation. Remember, babies are curious about everything and don't need much beyond normal domestic happenings to keep them busy. *Keep things simple.*

At the squirmer stage, your baby will start to have stability on her back (supine). With limbs bent, she will begin bringing her bib to her mouth. She will also discover her legs and eventually grasp her feet. While on her tummy (prone), she will begin to use elbow support, playing with toys with two hands and even shifting her weight to one elbow to grab for objects. By the end of this stage, some babies will start to roll from tummy to back or back to tummy!

Once baby can move his hands forward on his own, he will have more stability and easily move his head from side to side. He will follow external stimuli such as an adult walking past or a cat darting across the room. This stage builds his upper-body strength as well as head and eye coordination. Even at this young age, he is already using flexion and extension in a complex way. Chubby little arms are flexing while head and tail are extending.

Once baby has thoroughly explored stability on two arms, you can place a very simple toy close to him. At first he will bat at it with two hands. This is an important piece—he is establishing his center, so no need to rush him. Soon, he will shift his weight onto one arm, freeing up the other to reach for the toy. This stage lays the foundation for future writing, eating, instrument playing, painting—anything we do with one arm. When he gets to that point in school, he will need to stabilize with one hand while moving the other.

As adults, we tend to overlook the importance of the stabilizing arm, but both arms have important jobs. This is another example of the reptilian brain developing skills that will become automatic later in life. Being able to automatically stabilize with a helper hand while using a mover hand will free up your child's cortex to use advanced writing skills like decoding symbols, utilizing parts of speech, and assigning meaning. Older children who have not acquired the automatic use of a stabilizer arm and mobilizing arm can have trouble writing, throwing a ball, swimming, learning an instrument, knowing left from right, and even staying clean while they eat.

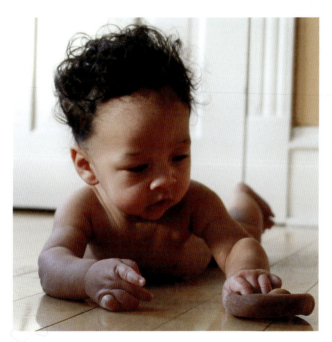

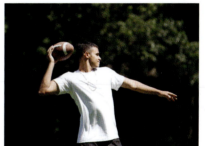

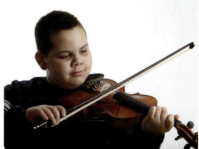

Nelson is stabilizing one arm by leaning on it; this frees up this other arm to grab a toy. This is a very important step in learning to eat, write, and throw a ball. His body is learning to do two separate tasks with each arm.

By practicing doing two separate tasks with each arm, babies prepare for more complicated tasks like throwing a ball or playing the violin.

Now We're Moving!

What if baby does not like to spend time on her tummy?

I get so many questions about what to do if baby fusses and cries when placed on her tummy. There are a few things we can try to make baby more comfortable on the tummy. First, try different times of day, experimenting with a full and less full tummy. Second, make sure tummy time doesn't also mean alone time—get on the floor with your baby and be close. Make sure baby is on a firm, flat surface. A surface that is too soft and squishy is hard to move on—imagine doing your workout on a water bed! And lastly, a baby needs to have developed some flexion strength along the front of the body to be comfortable on her tummy. This means her spine and limbs can soften into support and help her stabilize and grab toys. If you notice your baby's body in full extension, much like an airplane with arms and/or legs straight and hovering off the floor, there is a good chance she does not have the needed flexion strength to be comfortable on the tummy. Here is what you can try: have baby spend more time on her back with a simple toy. Gently press her legs into the hips and her arms toward the center of her body. Gentle but deep compression to the joints invites flexion to them and will contribute to more comfort on the tummy. If your baby's time on her back has typically been spent under a play gym, take that away. Time on the back is for developing flexion strength by bringing arms and legs into the body. Toys and balls dangling above baby cause baby to reach out for them and extend, extend, extend while reaching and kicking them. Best for baby to just be entertained with a small toy or object that she can actually hold and bring close to her to develop the flexion needed for successful time on the tummy. Babies born prematurely often do

> not have the flexion strength needed to bring their limbs into the center when laying on their backs. To build this flexion strength, these babies will benefit from lying on their sides rather than their backs.

What You Will See in the Squirmer Stage

Prone/On tummy:

- Hands coming together
- Holding head at ninety degrees while on her tummy
- Supporting herself on her forearms
- Shifting weight from one arm to the other
- Mouthing toys to investigate their texture
- Beginning to take weight on her hands
- Reaching with one arm
- Batting at and handling toys
- Maintaining better head control

Supine/On back:

- Feet coming together to touch
- Hands meeting knees
- Ankles coming together to touch
- Possibly beginning to roll from back to side
- Hands finding feet
- Two hands grabbing one foot
- Bringing feet to mouth
- Handling objects while on his side
- Maintaining better head control

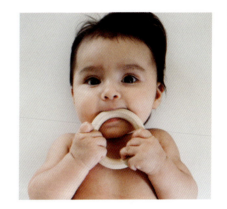

Luciana is finding her midline and practicing holding a toy with two hands. This type of circular toy is perfect for developing bilateral strength.

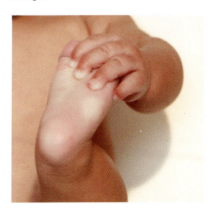

Now We're Moving!

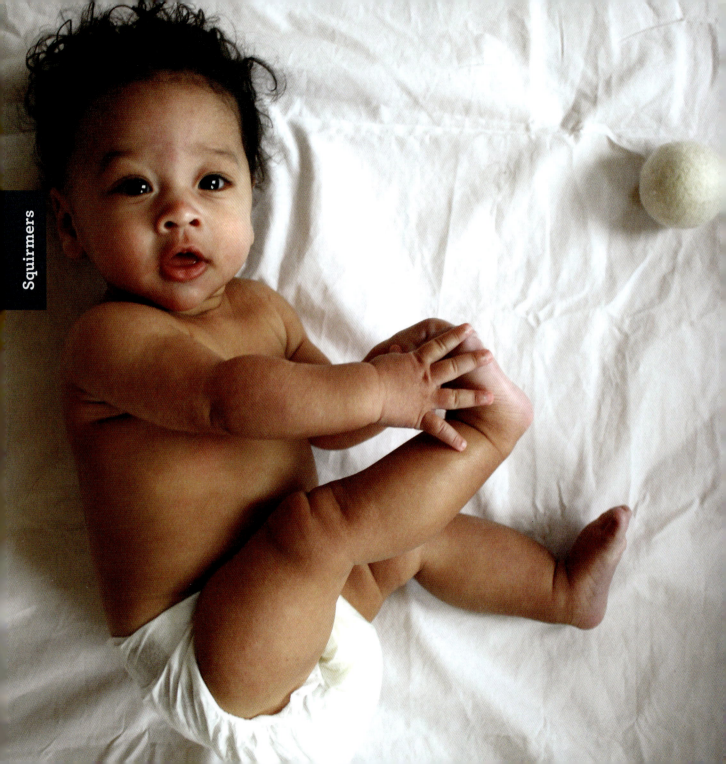
Squirmers

Ways to Support Baby's Squirmer Stage

- Allow plenty of time for unrestricted movement
- Apply deep but gentle pressure to baby's joints.
- Offer baby some diaper-free time. A good time for this would be after you have cleaned her soiled diaper. Watch closely and clean up any fecal matter that may sneak out during naked time. Also, make sure the temperature is nice and warm.
- Keep toys simple and light
- Alternate the hand you use to offer a toy, or put the toy on the floor next to baby
- Wear baby in a carrier rather than toting him around in a car seat. This is better for you and baby. While using a body carrier, be sure to wear baby facing inward.
- Expose baby to a variety of textures—warm and cold pieces of fruit, rough and smooth toys, and so on. Gently move the object all over baby's body and let him feel the sensation, naming the texture while he experiences them.

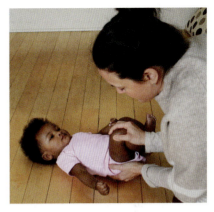

Luca will be able to play on her tummy with more joy and ease if she receives frequent pressure to her hips and shoulders. Press firmly and gently; watch your baby's face, she will let you know if she doesn't like it. She may not be in the mood or you may be pressing to hard; if this happens, back off a bit and/or try again later.

Being close is still very important for your baby; you will find she is better able to play and explore with you nearby.

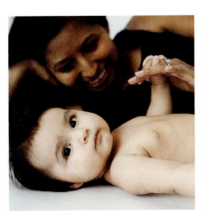
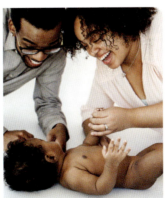
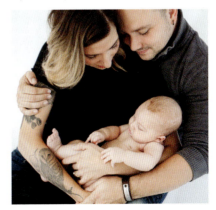

Now We're Moving!

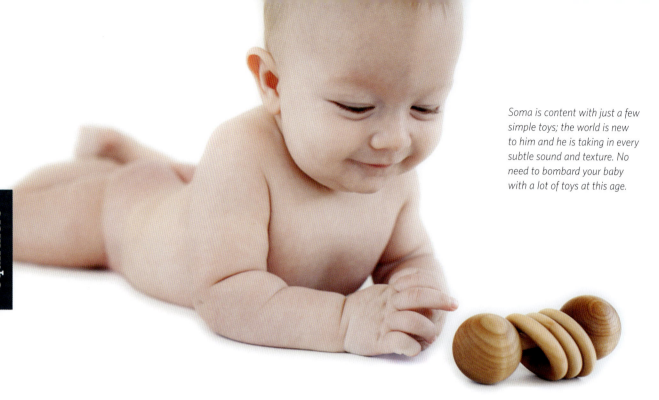

Soma is content with just a few simple toys; the world is new to him and he is taking in every subtle sound and texture. No need to bombard your baby with a lot of toys at this age.

- Sing to baby—nursery rhymes and lullabies are great, but if you don't know any, sing your favorite songs. Don't worry about having a "good" voice. Your voice is music to your baby's ears, and singing can be calming for both of you.
- Swing, rock, sway, cuddle—be in contact with your baby as much as you can throughout the day
- Feed on both sides and hold baby while bottle-feeding
- Attend to baby's cries
- Stay close—baby loves to have you down on the floor with her while she plays
- When baby is supine, start to offer him toys after he has started playing with his bib
- Place baby on his tummy without bringing arms forward for him. He will eventually move them forward on his own.

What to Avoid in the Squirmer Stage

- Avoid hanging toys above your baby. She will want to bring them to her mouth for exploration. If she can't reach them, she'll just hit and kick them, which could interfere with the development of balance between flexion and extension. If the toy is above her, she will likely just be reaching and reaching, overusing her extensor muscles but never really flexing and bringing objects in toward her for closer inspection.
- Don't encourage baby to sit. Keep her in a horizontal position as much as possible unless you are holding or wearing her.
- Don't leave baby in a car seat unless you are traveling
- Don't stand baby up
- Don't teach her to move forward on her tummy or place toys so far away that she needs to move forward to get them
- Don't roll her over
- Don't pull her up by the hands to a sitting position
- Don't bring her arms forward while in a prone position
- Keep your baby away from all media and television. For more on this, see "Protect Your Baby from Overpowering Stimulus" in chapter 4.
- Avoid letting baby cry or feel frustrated for too long. Babies need you to teach them to self-soothe. The more you soothe your upset baby, the more familiar she is with the feeling of being calm and will be able to find it on her own eventually. If she is not soothed by you, the feeling of calm and recovery from feeling upset is unfamiliar to her and it will be difficult to recreate on her own when she is older. Rock a crying baby, sing to her, or simply hold her close.

. . . .

Now We're Moving!

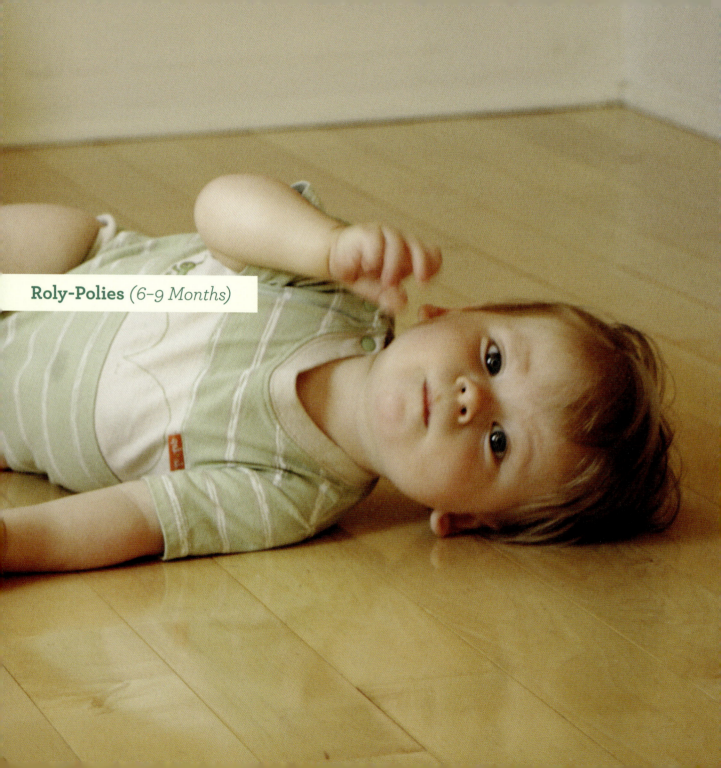

Roly-Polies *(6-9 Months)*

During this stage, you will see your baby become more mobile. Rolling and exploring front, back, and side playing are all ways baby prepares for the lizard crawl. This stage is very important as it sets the foundation for crawling and creeping. Some babies will begin to push up to sitting during this stage and others will do that during the next stage of crawling. Remember that it is important to let your baby find her own way to sitting and there is no rush.

Baby will begin the joys of rolling! At first she may roll from back to front, often looking a bit surprised by this big shift in perspective the first few times it happens! Baby is using one side to hoist herself over, while she presses her other side into the floor. She is learning to accomplish two separate functions on each side of her body. Rolling requires stabilizing one side while the other side works. Later in the crawling stage, this ability will evolve into being able to flex one side while extending the other.

Soon baby will be rolling from front to back and back to front as a method of locomotion. It is important that he can roll to both left and right sides. This ensures that he will develop equal strength on both sides. Rolling to both sides is necessary to reach another landmark, often called a "milestone"—sitting independently. While you may be tempted to prop your baby up to teach him to sit, please know that by accomplishing the roll on both sides, your baby is building the strength to sit on his own when the time is right. Some babies will begin to explore this with their rolling and others will wait until they have some experience with lizard crawling. Getting into the sitting position from the floor is very complex and something we want baby to learn for himself. Sometimes to understand the difficulty of a movement your baby is doing, it is helpful to try it out in your own body. From your tummy, experiment with ways to get to sitting. Slow it down and really feel all the components that are at work to orchestrate the shift from tummy to sitting. This is not something we want baby to skip—there's so much good work to be done!

Many of the movements you will see your baby do—rolling, spending time on his side as he brings his hand or a toy to his mouth—help develop his

Roly-Polies

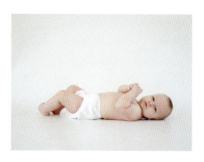
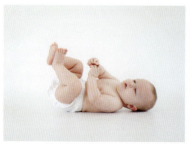
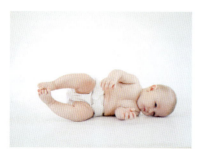
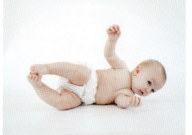
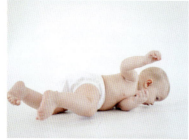
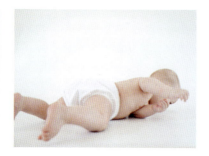
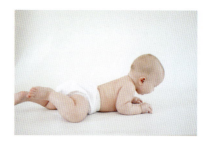

midline. Establishing his midline will be absolutely crucial for reading and problem-solving throughout his life. We will say much more about this in the section on the creeper stage.

Baby will start to push himself up to sit on his rear end. It is important for you to resist the urge to sit him up and expect him to find his own balance. Allow him to move through this stage and find his own way to sitting. When babies are made to sit up or put in devices that hold them up before they are ready, their legs and hips often have to brace or remain in extension to hold up their bodies. This makes moving from sitting to crawling to sitting again very difficult. This is a great example of how a balance of flexion and extension becomes functional and allows a child to mobilize through the world with ease. A baby who is propped up does not have the same ease of motion and

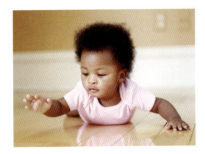
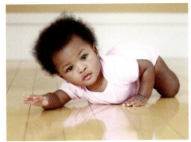

Luca is learning to roll from front to back; lying on her back gives her a whole new perspective and soon she will be able to roll back and forth depending on how she wants to play. It's important that she rolls to her right and left side to develop the strength needed for sitting and crawling in a few months!

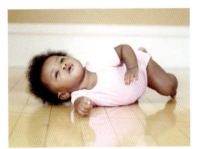
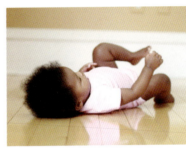

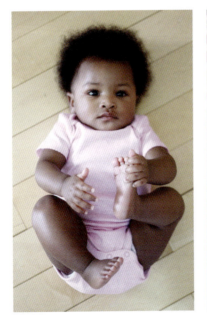
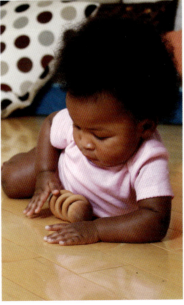

Luca has plenty of flexion strength, making it easy and enjoyable to explore playing with toys on her side.

Now We're Moving!

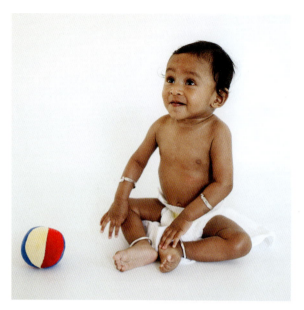

Shayan is just getting comfortable with sitting. Once he gets a bit stronger he will be able to play with toys in the sitting position; that requires a strong lower body so the arms can be free to play, just like drawing, writing, playing the piano, and any task in the sitting position.

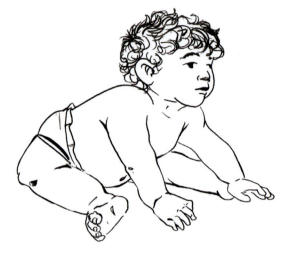

This baby is not ready to sit yet. He is leaning forward, causing his hips and lower back to brace in order to hold himself up. When babies are allowed to find their way to sitting, we can be certain that they have the underlying support to sit upright while hips and back are free to move and fold rather than just brace stiffly. Avoid propping baby up in a foam seat or any other device that encourages sitting before baby can get herself to sitting unassisted.

will have to rely on stiff straight legs and hips to keep himself up. It's hard to move with stiff legs!

Sitting will become more stable with practice. Once your baby gets some practice getting to the sitting position, you will see him next be able to hold things and play with his hands, clap his hands together. This shows that the lower body is sturdy and strong and can support baby while his hands and arms get busy with simple toys, clapping, and joyously moving when he hears music. A great sitter is one who can move rather than just sit braced in the position. Your baby will eventually learn to shift from sitting to all fours and back, and to reach for a toy and find his way back to sitting to play with it.

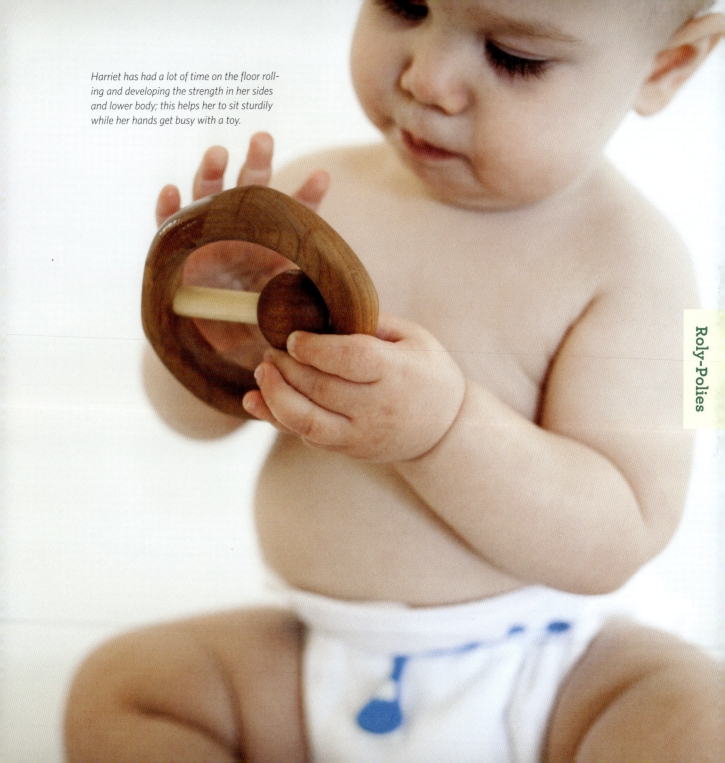

Harriet has had a lot of time on the floor rolling and developing the strength in her sides and lower body; this helps her to sit sturdily while her hands get busy with a toy.

Roly-Polies

This shifting from sitting to reaching and taking weight on the hands back to sitting is complex and well worth every minute your baby spends working on it. Remember back to when your baby was just opening and closing the limbs as one unit. Now watch how he folds one leg under and pushes through it while reaching for a toy and coming back to sitting with it in his hand. So much has been learned; this will all serve him throughout his life. This time navigating the world on the floor is priceless and we have such a short window for it. Sit back and allow it to happen—before you know it he will be riding a bike and doing calculus. Enjoy watching this; enjoy every minute of it.

The Roly-Poly stage is crucial for developing a sense of the midline. Baby does this by exploring her weight against gravity in a variety of angles and planes on the floor. Awareness of their midline also enables babies to creep on all fours, an exciting time for all new parents. We are often eager to see baby get to creeping on all fours because we recognize it as a milestone of development. Please remember that everything baby does before creeping is developing the right muscle coordination and awareness to fully engage in creeping.

What You Will See in the Roly-Poly Stage

- Baby is establishing his midline or sense of center. Once established, he will be able to cross it later for things like reading, problem-solving, skipping, and tying shoes.
- Core strength development, which will help baby sit up later on and establish a foundation for muscle development, body composition, and tone.
- Awareness of the different sides of his body, along with the ability to do separate tasks with each side, will allow him to stabilize one side of the body while the other one moves when he's older.

Something to think about...

Your baby is doing very hard work as she explores these stages of development. Sometimes she will get fussy or frustrated. While we never want to allow a baby to get too upset while playing on the floor, we also want to avoid swiftly picking baby up with every peep she makes. I do recommend attending and interacting with baby when she vocalizes. As baby grows, her range of communication expands and you will begin to recognize the subtle differences in the sounds she makes. Sometimes when a baby is working hard, she can vocalize a grunt or two. When this occurs, I suggest you get down on the floor with your baby and acknowledge the hard work.

"This is really a struggle. I see you are working so hard." Give your baby some time to work hard before picking her up. You might sense that she is done and needs a break. "That's enough for now; we'll try again later." Offer a change of scenery and hold her for a while. Again, we do not want baby to get too upset, but we also don't want to rescue her from her hard work too soon. I work with many parents who pick up baby at every little peep they hear. As baby gets older, her communication will become more diverse. Although it's important to attend to every cry, it is equally as important to become familiar with your baby's expanding range of communication.

- Baby will roll from tummy to back in both directions, left and right. Baby will also roll from back to tummy in both directions during this stage. You will see him rest in the middle on his side often; this is all part of his work.

Ways to Support Baby's Roly-Poly Stage

- Provide ample time on the floor
- Find a smooth surface so baby can push and pull on the floor. Try not to cover his feet in socks or tights that might cause him to slip.
- Take diapers off when possible. It is much easier for baby to flex at the hips without that bulky diaper.
- Sing to baby and play music. Music made by instruments and/or LP records is best for baby's development (digital recordings are fine, too). Playing music from around the world exposes baby to a variety of sounds.
- Swing, rock, waltz, gallop, skip, walk, and run while holding baby. Freeze once in a while to help baby develop his vestibular system (his sense of where his body is located in space).
- Go outside with baby. There are so many sights, sounds, and smells for baby to explore outside. Let baby feel grass, sand, dirt, leaves, flowers, water, and so on. Be alert to baby putting things in his mouth—not all grass is chemical free! When baby tries to put things in his mouth (and he will), gently say, "Just for hands and feet," while you put some grass or sand on his feet. We want to encourage a range of sensory exploration, but also need to watch very closely, as babies will try to "explore" with their mouths.
- Read aloud to baby. Rhyming books and nursery rhymes are best, but if you need a break, reading a few pages from your summer novel or a cookbook is fine, too. The vibration of your voice stimulates baby's vocal chords for his own language development.

- Label things for baby: "This is a book," "The grass is prickly," "The water is cool," and so on. Avoid asking baby, "Is the water cool?" "Is the grass prickly?" "Is this a book?"
- Offer simple toys with different shapes and textures. Household objects like measuring cups and spoons provide a safe and interesting variety. After all, we want baby to learn about his environment, and his home is his first classroom. Fancy toys that light up and make sounds are not suitable for brain development. They also do not help baby learn about the domestic setting and rhythms of home. Home is the most interesting place to a baby; let him explore it.

What to Avoid in the Roly-Poly Stage

- Do not sit baby up. He will learn to do this on his own if he is allowed to explore through movement.
- Do not stand baby up or teach walking and crawling. The movements and time that he spends getting there are very important for physical, emotional, and cognitive development.
- Use car seat for traveling only
- Protect baby from inappropriate sounds and stimuli: loud music, a cacophony of background sounds, television, harsh chemicals, crying too long without soothing support, and so on
- Avoid use of devices that restrict movement. When you need to ensure baby's safety, use room gates to section off a safe area to explore.

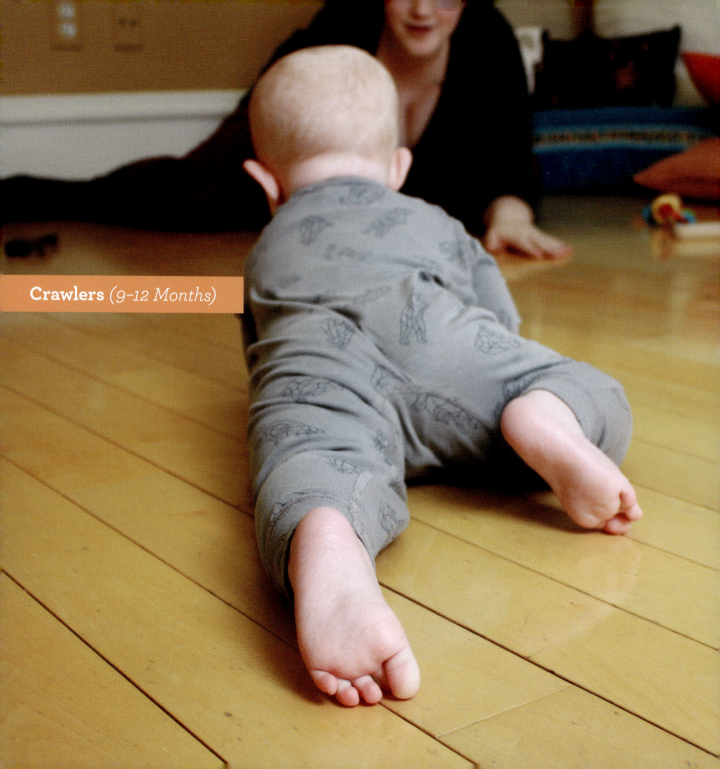

Crawlers *(9-12 Months)*

Everything baby has done on the floor thus far—rolling, pushing, pulling, pivoting, and so on—has prepared her for this stage of locomotion. This crawling stage is sometimes referred to as belly crawling or lizard crawling. It is different from how we typically imagine crawling, which is on all fours, but in this book, we will call that more commonly thought-of movement creeping.

In my clinical practice, this is probably the stage I see most often skipped by children of well-meaning parents. In this important stage, many of the previously learned skills are coming together with increased complexity. She will crawl across the floor in this way, watching her extended hand as she moves. While she watches the thumb of that extended hand, she is actually developing something called **horizontal eye tracking**. Horizontal eye tracking, or moving your eyes from side to side, is essential to reading later in life. By watching each hand as it extends while she moves, she automatically builds the ability to move her eyes from side to side.

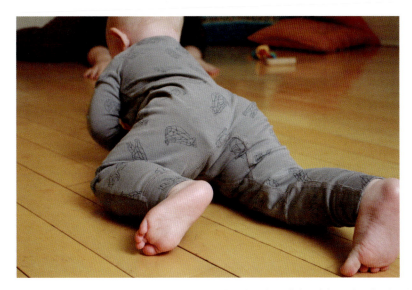
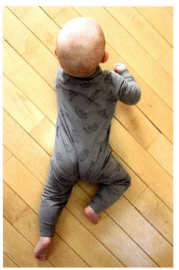

Juniper is flexing one side of her body while extending the other, all the while tracking her hands as she moves through the room. This is crucial for preparing her body and brain for future reading, writing, and complex tasks like throwing and playing an instrument.

Now We're Moving!

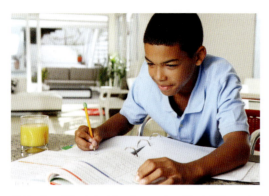

Notice how this student is using one hand to stabilize and the other to move his pencil? This is a complex skill; since it was practiced during infancy, it is automatic for him and his cortex can focus on grammar, spelling, and composition.

Remember, everything learned on the floor becomes automatic and a function of the hindbrain. The movement of the eyes while we are reading needs to be automatic to free the cortex for the other tasks of reading.

Lizard crawling is also crucial to further developing a stabilizing hand and a moving hand, which we know baby will need to write. Later in life, her body will automatically understand that it can do two different things at once—flexion on one side and extension on the other—or stabilize one side while mobilizing the other.

What You Will See in the Crawling Stage

- The crawling stage often begins with baby pushing backwards with two arms. This seems counterproductive to us because we have visions of baby moving forward toward something. Why would they move back? Moving backwards requires a strong push with the upper body. Their shoulders, arms, hands, and back are building strength.
- After a period of pushing back, baby will start to pivot around in a circular motion. Watch this pivoting action; it is typically with one hand working at a time, often one hand crossing over the other. This is more complex than the pushing backward—the one-handed pivot is the next step after the two-handed push back. Now we can see why the push back was so important—it takes strength to pivot one hand at a time!
- Lastly, you will see baby move forward with belly on the floor like a lizard. This often begins during a pivot: one chubby little bare foot at the end of a bent leg will feel the floor and push against it. This little push propels baby forward, and soon those little legs and feet will be positioning up and down pushing baby forward.

What the world may tell you about belly crawling...

When my son August was nine months old, he was doing a beautiful, textbook-perfect lizard crawl, and I knew it was exactly what he should be doing at that stage. I brought him to the local recreational center for a class for children ages zero to three—one of those experiential music classes in which you and your child play with instruments or large multi-colored parachutes, etc. One day during this class, the teacher dumped a pile of toys out in the center of the room and called out that all the children could come and get one. So, August crawled over on his belly, got a toy, and brought it back to me. There happened to be a lovely elderly woman next to me who was taking the class with her granddaughter. She saw August crawl across the floor on his belly and looked up at me. I will never forget the expression on her face. It was filled with sympathetic pity and concern. Then she smiled gently and said in her most assuring tone, "Don't worry, honey. He'll be walking soon."

This story illustrates just how misinformed our society has become about what babies need. By crawling across the floor on his belly, August was doing exactly what he was developmentally supposed to be doing. He was building the mechanisms in his hindbrain that would serve him later in life. But, in the eyes of this well-meaning stranger, here was a child who was moving in a way that seemed strange and therefore wrong to her. We have become so intent on speeding through developmental movement stages, with the idea that sooner is better when it comes to walking, that it's almost as if we look upon anything that happens on the

Continued on next page

floor as primitive or animalistic. This kindly grandmother was just trying to comfort and assure me that my son would eventually "grow out" of his lizard crawling, as though it were something to be concerned about. But, as a clinician, I have seen firsthand the difficulties and delays children who speed through or skip this stage struggle with later in life.

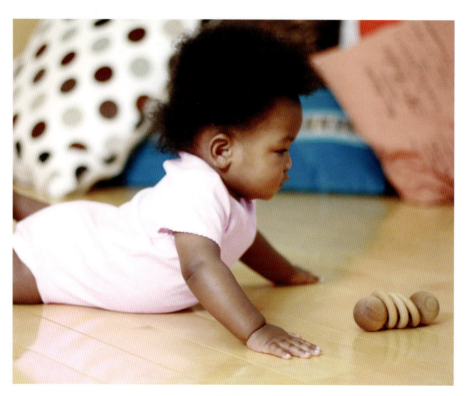

Luca is pushing back with her upper body. This is the first step to belly crawling; she is gaining the necessary strength to eventually go forward. Try placing toys behind her as it will be frustrating to have toys in front of her that she can't get to yet.

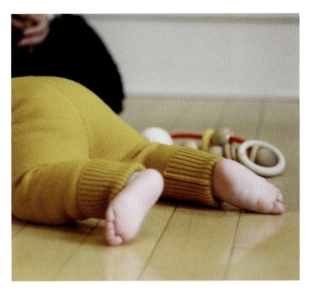
Elias is pivoting around himself exploring what he can reach this way. He is preparing his upper and lower body to work together in the full belly crawl that will happen soon. He is also moving his arms one at a time, all preparing him for moving forward on his tummy.

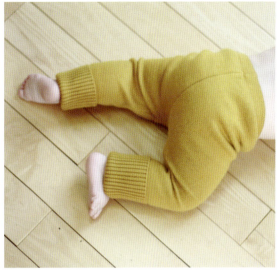
When Elias feels the floor under that foot, he will push into the floor and propel himself forward.

- Each method of locomoting on the floor allows baby plenty of opportunity to visually track his hands with his eyes. Watching his own hands from this position assures that his eyes will be horizontally tracking automatically—this is crucial for reading and writing throughout life. This is not a stage to rush—100 percent of the school-aged children in my practice did not lizard crawl during infancy.
- Many babies begin pushing themselves up to sitting in this stage. With the increased folding and flexing of the lower body and strengthening of the sides with the belly crawling, the body is really primed to push arms into the floor, tuck legs under, and reach the bottom back to sit. While some babies do start this during the Roly-Poly stage, it is often because parents are propping them up to "teach" sitting.

Juniper is on her way now! This pushing against the floor with her feet is building core strength and wiring her lower body for speed, strength, and optimal alignment.

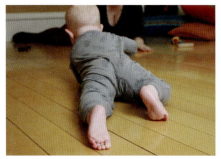
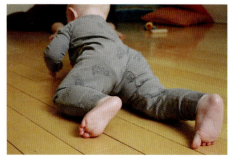

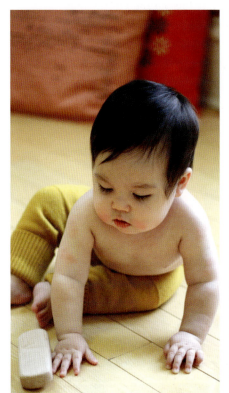

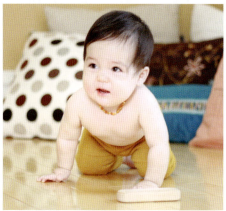

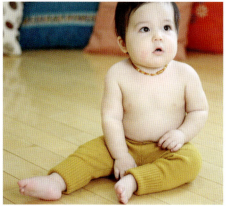

Elias is finding his way to the sitting position. By pushing and extending his arms while folding and flexing his legs, he is learning to do two separate tasks with the top and bottom of his body. This will help him sit still in a chair and eat, write, draw, or play the piano.

Something to think about...

Now that baby is able to crawl around the room, you will need to practice some redirection skills. You will begin to use your voice and face to let baby know what is okay and what is not. Stay calm, firm, and consistent. Baby will be confused if you laugh while redirecting him from exploring something hot. He needs to see your whole body commit to the directive. For example, say, "This is dangerous," with a firm tone and neutral but serious face. I often coach parents to save the word "no" for things that baby can never touch, such as cords, electrical outlets, the stove, dog food dish, etc. Find another way to redirect when baby is exploring something that is appropriate for bigger people but not for babies, such as the remote control, phone, delicate decorations, etc. "That's not for baby" or "Let's just look with our eyes" while you hold onto it, is appropriate. You may also offer another interesting object while taking one way and saying, "I have this, too."

As baby begins to be more mobile, avoid using "No, no" all day long to keep baby safe. Start by making sure baby's space is safe. When you do need to redirect baby, tell him what you are doing and simply state, "That's not for baby." For example, if baby is crawling toward the television cords, you may say, "I'm going to move you now to keep you safe. That's not for babies." Interrupting baby constantly with "no" may give the impression that his world is not safe to explore. We also want to avoid teaching patterns of interruption vs. patterns of completion. When a baby motors towards an object, it's important he be able to complete the cycle: see it, motor toward it, and touch it or put it into his mouth and explore it. If baby moves toward something that he can explore with his hands and eyes but not his mouth, oversee and guide his exploration rather than just saying "no."

If your baby's feet are not finding the floor to dig in, you may push gently but firmly into the flexed leg. This will encourage her to push against you and help her learn to push the floor for her belly crawling.

Crawlers

Ways to Support Baby's Crawling Stage

- Keep baby's feet bare. Prior to this forward crawling, your baby most likely was pushing herself backwards. A bare foot will help her feet feel the floor, and she will dig that fat little foot into the floor and realize she can propel herself forward. If she has socks, booties, or tights on, she will slip and slide and be more likely to skip this stage and prematurely go to creeping.
- Place baby on a smooth surface. Carpet will act like Velcro and make it too difficult to crawl on the belly. This may cause baby to skip this stage and go straight to creeping.
- Get down on the floor with baby
- Have a few simple toys or interesting objects for her to travel to, grab, and explore
- Balls are great for this stage. You can roll one a few feet from baby and she will delight in crawling after it. Let her grab and explore before you roll again. For babies there is such delight and reward in traveling to the object and playing with it.
- Sing and read to your baby. Simple nursery rhymes and books are great.
- Swing, dance, gallop, skip, and twirl with your baby
- Wear a sling or baby carrier when going on outings. Remember to keep baby facing in rather than out.

What to Avoid in the Crawling Stage

- Don't teach baby to creep or walk
- Don't place baby in a Jolly Jumper, Bumbo, ExerSaucer, or swings
- Protect baby from media and other inappropriate stimuli
- Don't put baby in car seat unless you are traveling

Now We're Moving!

- Avoid interrupting baby when she is exploring. If you must interrupt to keep her safe, simply tell her what you are doing. Often a baby's movements are inspired by a desire to look at something more closely, feel it, or put it in her mouth. We want to encourage habits of completion as often as possible. Constantly being interrupted can enforce habits of interruption, which is not optimal.

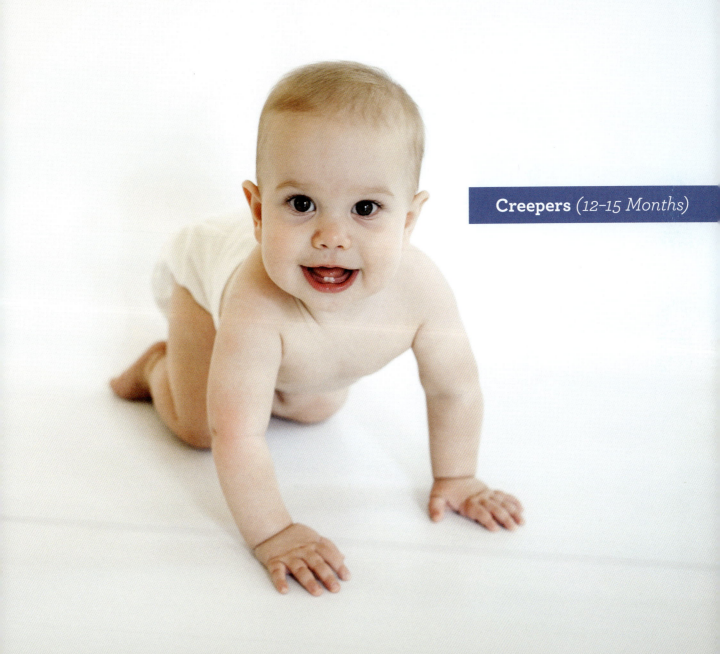

Creepers *(12–15 Months)*

Hooray! We've made it to creeping across the floor on all fours! In this stage we see the first evidence of crosslateral movement. Crosslateral movement is opposite diagonal movement, in that one arm and the opposite leg stabilize while the other arm and opposite leg move. Thus, opposite sides are flexing and extending. This ability is crucial to all kinds of future skills, like walking and running. This crosslateral movement shows that the hemispheres of the brain are integrating. Hemisphere integration is crucial for reading, physical coordination, and problem-solving. Also, the two sides of the body are working together; the upper and lower body are working together; the head and tail or spine is strong and integrated; the neck is strong and integrated; and the eyes can look out ahead and move independently.

This is the stage parents and grandparents really seem to resonate with. We are accustomed to seeing baby's locomote this way, and we see these images in the media most frequently. I can't tell you how many times parents have asked me, "When will my baby crawl for real?" While I can sense the enthusiasm these parents have to see their baby do what is familiar to them, it also serves as an invitation to educate them about the important steps that prepare babies to "crawl for real," or creep, as we call this stage.

When your baby is ready to creep, you might first see her rock back and forth on hands and knees as if she is revving up her engine. She is actually preparing to move on all fours. She will look down at the floor and back up at her mom or dad, then down at the floor and up at the dog, and so on. This ability to focus near and far will help her in all kinds of ways, such as when she looks down at her desk and then up at a teacher. In addition, drawing a distinction between her upper and lower body will help her sit still while her arms and head work. In the same way that rolling develops right and left sides, this revving up solidifies the ability to separate two tasks between the lower and upper body. The lower body is flexing and the upper body is extending.

Elias just found his weight on his arms!

Creepers

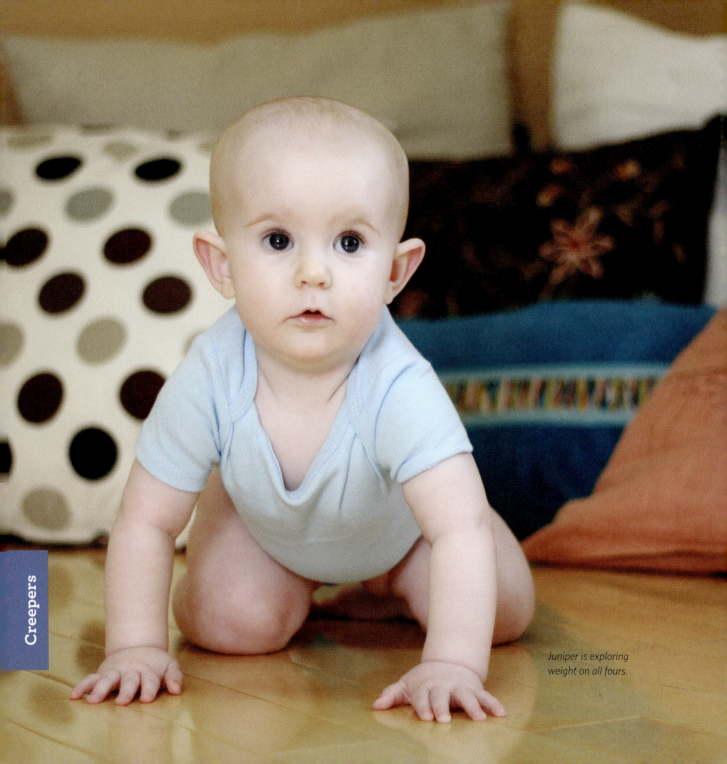

Creepers

Juniper is exploring weight on all fours.

Revving up establishes that baby can do two different things with the upper and lower halves of her body. She will demonstrate flexion in her legs and extension in her torso, back, and arms. She will need this ability later in life when she has to sit in a chair, thus stabilizing her lower body while she moves her upper body.

Baby's first efforts will be a bit rougher than they will be at the end of this stage; she will take some time to figure out how to alternate and shift weight throughout her body to move forward. This is where all that core strength she developed in previous stages will come in handy. Her center is strong and can provide stability while her arms and legs explore alternating weight bearing and moving on this new level. She will eventually move forward and backward with a smoother rhythm and also easily go from sitting to creeping to explore her world. You will also begin to see stair climbing and bear walking with just feet and hands on the floor and hips raised up to the ceiling. All these movements are a true culmination of everything baby has developed so far.

Once baby can creep so fast that she beats you to the door or a toy, you know she is ready to walk. Keep in mind that between twelve and fifteen months is a perfectly fine time to start walking. As I'm sure you know by now, there is no reason to rush to teach baby to walk.

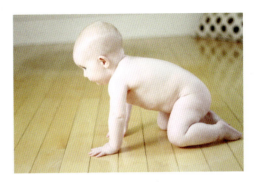

Juniper is revving up; this helps her get used to transferring weight between her arms and legs. Soon, she will take her first creeping steps!

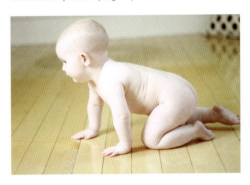

And Juniper is off!

Now We're Moving!

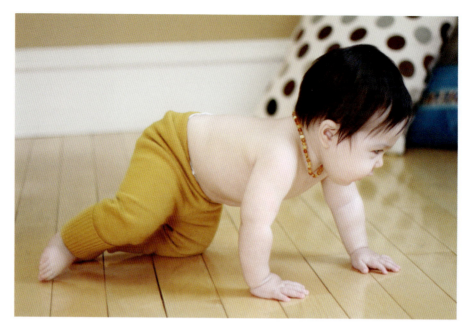

Elias taking his first creeping steps; these will be cautious and will get more confident and smooth as he practices.

What You Will See in the Creeper Stage

- Baby will begin the stage by bouncing on her hands and knees back and forth. This is needed for all sorts of activities that require upper-lower coordination, including driving, writing, running, tennis, painting, playing piano, making a model airplane, eating, etc.
- Slowly baby will begin to make an effort to take weight on hands and knees and travel forward. This will be hard and slow at first; remember, something new is happening here. Left and right are working in a new way. The opposite arm and leg are taking weight while the other lifts.
- This is the culmination of all the other stages, and will allow baby mobility in the body and hemisphere integration in the neocortex.

Mac is on the go—no stopping him now! By spending plenty of time exploring his world on all fours, he is integrating his brain hemispheres for reading and problem-solving just to name a couple.

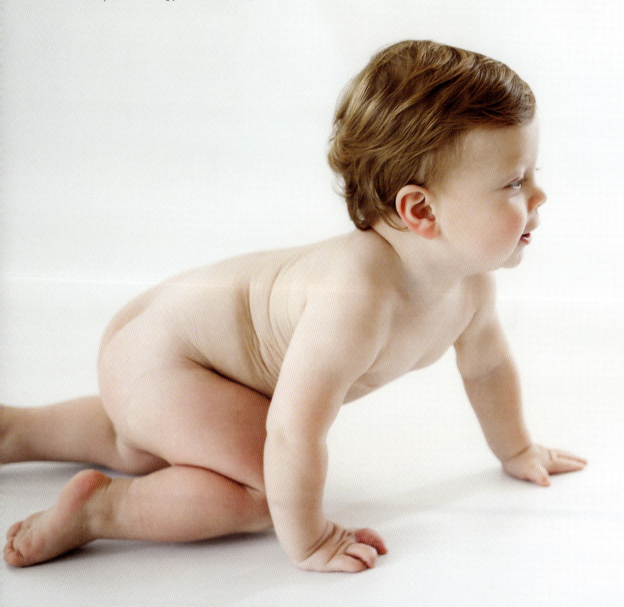

Creepers

Mac can now flex and extend with ease because he was given all the time he needed to developed through each stage at his own time. Thanks for not rushing me, Mom!

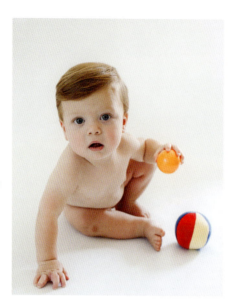
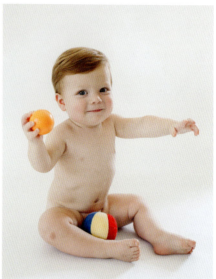

- You will see baby move with ease from sitting to crawling to get toys and explore
- Baby now has many ways to move through the room. You may see her use all of them, alternating between rolling, crawling, and creeping.

Ways to Support Baby's Creeper Stage

- Prepare the space. Keep large areas of your home clear for movement exploration. You may want to move coffee tables and ottomans out of the main play space for this period if you have not already. We want to encourage as much floor time as possible. Too many things to pull up on will interfere with your baby's floor time.
- Provide many types of movement opportunities, inside and outside your home. Some children may be ready for a regular playgroup, and you may really enjoy some time with other parents.

- Get on the floor with your child
- Swing, skip, dance, rock, and sway your baby
- Listen to and create music with your baby
- Label objects in the home without quizzing baby: "This is Mommy's scarf."
- Reflect your baby's sounds and emotions
- Use safety gates to keep baby from areas you do not want him to explore without an adult

Something to think about...

As your baby starts moving more and more, you will have the opportunity to create balance between hovering over every move she makes and providing too little supervision. We all are aware of the term "helicopter parent," used to describe that parent at the park who hovers over his or her child's every move. Only *you* know your child's areas of strength and development. If you feel like hovering is what your child needs while he finds his footing at the park, then do that. As you see your child accomplish more and more, you will continue to adjust your level of "hovering" accordingly. Some children are very timid and may need your encouragement and help to try new things; others show no fear and need to be watched while they learn what is safe. While it is instinctive to protect our children from every bump and bruise, it's important to remember that small tumbles and run-ins with slippery slides are part of your child's way of figuring out his body, his limits, and his world. More important than preventing such tumbles is to console, soothe, rub "owies," and encourage children to keep playing when these inevitable small tumbles occur.

What to Be Aware of in the Creeper Stage

- Avoid teaching your child to walk
- Avoid using walking assistants like little shopping carts or other toys that baby can lean on to help her walk
- Use car seats only for traveling
- Protect baby from media and other inappropriate stimuli
- Do not use devices (swings, chairs, play-gyms, etc.) designed for aiding your baby in bouncing, sitting, or walking. Your baby's unencumbered movement is more than enough at this stage.
- Do not interrupt baby. If you must to keep her safe, simply tell her what you are doing: "Mom is going to move you away for safety." We want to create patterns of completion rather than interruption.

All the work that your baby has done up until now has led her to this point. She has developed all the skills necessary to accomplish this beautiful task. And by allowing her to develop her body, she has built a stronger brain from the bottom up. Congratulations!

. . . .

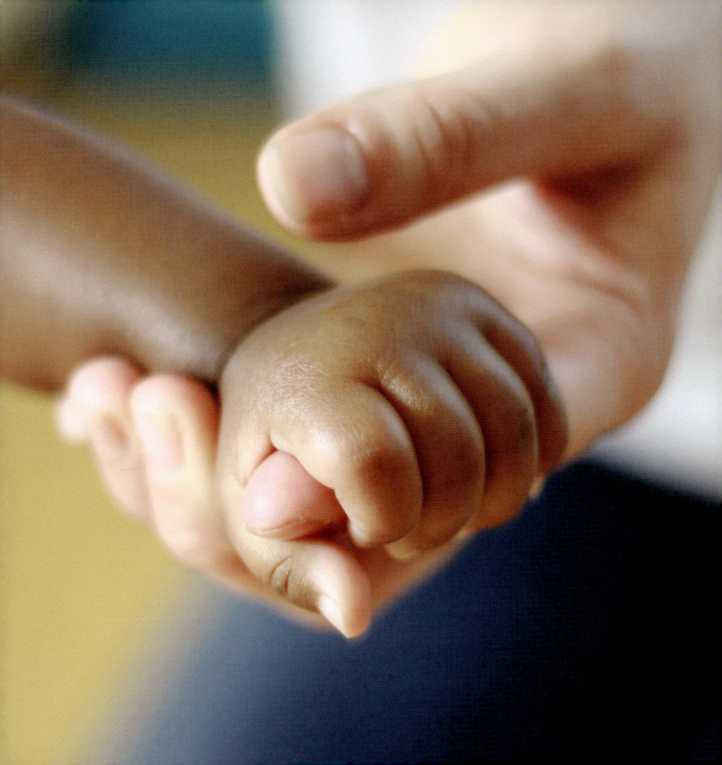

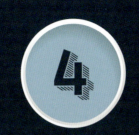

Social-Emotional Development

The Nervous System

Everything we have talked about so far in this book—the human brain and body, voluntary and involuntary movements—is part of a larger network we call the nervous system. The human nervous system, like all systems in nature, functions best when it is in balance. Think of yourself, for example—don't you feel most calm, centered, and happy when your life is in balance? How many of us have thought, "If only I could achieve more *balance*"? Yet too often, our hectic modern lives throw our nervous systems out of whack, and we feel stressed, overly stimulated, or just plain exhausted.

Let's revisit the concept of flexion and extension through a different lens, a social-emotional lens. Earlier in this book, we learned that flexion is the folding of the body's joints and limbs in toward the center of the body, while extension is the opening or extending of the joints and limbs away from the center of the body.

I want you to think of a time when you were scared for your life, perhaps when you were at the top of a giant roller coaster that you were dared to ride, or slamming on the breaks to avoid a car accident. Using our movement fundamentals of extension and flexion, what does our body do during these times of perceived threat?

Close your eyes and imagine yourself in a threatening situation: what do you feel your body doing? For most of us, we extend and brace our limbs, especially through the spine. The act of arching/extending the spine is paired with what we call the sympathetic nervous system (SNS). The SNS is also activated when we are excited; a healthy expression of the SNS would be seen when playing peek-a-boo, or when happy to be seeing a friend or animal at the zoo. It's important to remember that excited play is a natural function of the SNS and is a healthy and important part of development. However, sometimes the SNS is over-activated and the excitement is too much for the body to tolerate. This over-activated level is not optimal, and we will talk about why and how to avoid it. When the SNS is activated as a response to a threat, our body produces adrenaline and other stress hormones that are released by the adrenal glands, which sit right above the kidneys at our lower back. Our bodies are designed to release adrenaline and other stress hormones during times of perceived threat; doing so puts our body in alert mode, which helps keep us safe. The act of arching the body to squeeze those glands in our lower back is part of this system.

Now keep in mind that during threats and scares, when the body is on alert, all of our resources go to the hindbrain, which is our survival center and the home of all things automatic. When the SNS is activated, we become very aware of our surroundings in terms of exits and planning escape routes. Our pupils dilate to let in more light (to better assess the situation), and blood rushes to either our upper body for fighting or our lower body for running, depending on the nature of the threat. Heart regulation and breathing also change; breathing often becomes very shallow to preserve energy and/or avoid detection (think of a little rabbit barely breathing in hopes you don't see him). While it's true that the body prepares for threat in a variety of ways depending on the situation, extension is almost always a part of SNS activation.

The recuperative state of the SNS is the parasympathetic nervous system (PNS); this is the part that brings us back to calm regulation. Think of yourself after a nice bath or spooning with your mate, or how you feel after hugging the world's best hugger. Go ahead and imagine a time when you felt loved, well fed, well rested, and certain you were safe and had everything you needed. How does your body feel? For most of us, our limbs will be relaxed and easily folded into the body. Think of our language around calming activities, "*curling up* with a cup of tea," "*settling in* for the night." The body naturally goes inward (as in flexion) for calming. Just as extension is paired with the SNS, flexion is paired with the PNS.

There is a beautiful series of glands that runs down the front midline of the body that activates the PNS. By folding into the center, we massage the glands that help bring calm to our bodies. For those of you who practice yoga, think of poses that curl in and calm (such as child's pose) versus those that open and activate (camel pose and other back bends).

The SNS and the PNS are both important parts of our nervous system; neither is better than the other. SNS arousal is not bad; we just need to be aware of over activating it as it is expensive on the body's resources. Ideally, the SNS is only activated when we really are in danger. We are not meant to be leading our lives from a state of SNS arousal every day; to do so is very taxing on the nervous system. The key is to achieve balance, allowing your SNS and PNS to work in harmony with the body as needed.

Flexion and Extension: Finding the Balance

Let's get back to thinking about your baby's movement development. Earlier we learned that a balance of flexion and extension will ensure your baby can experience all the movements she is designed to go through. Essentially, the basic alphabet for all movements we do is flexing and extending various parts to execute increasingly complicated tasks. This balance is especially important to little bodies as they figure out how to move and navigate through this new world of theirs.

Beyond physical function and everyday tasks, the balance of flexion and extension in early development also has a very important role in the social and emotional development of your baby. Remember that during these months on the floor, we are wiring the hindbrain, the seat of all things automatic. Just as horizontal eye tracking becomes automatic and unconscious, so does our social-emotional relationship with our world. And it all develops here on the floor and in your arms.

Sometimes babies come in to my office and I notice their bodies are already favoring extension (meaning they typically arch their backs and their little legs and arms might be straight and stiff). In these cases, I'm not just

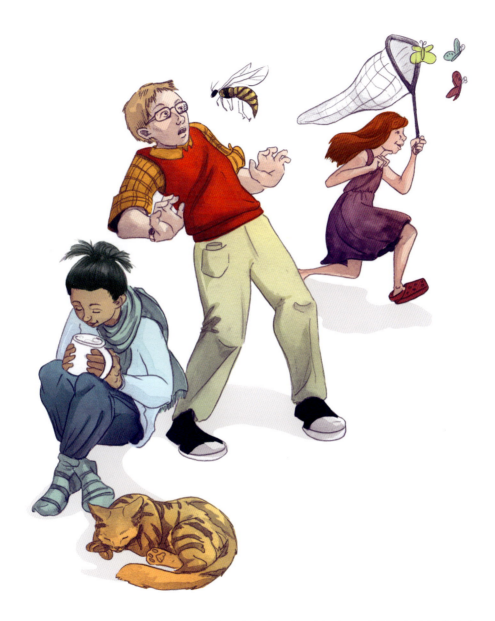

The balance of flexion and extension is also important for social and emotional development. Extension is implicated in the Sympathetic Nervous System (SNS) and flexion is paired with the Parasympathetic Nervous System (PNS).

> baby's system is very immature at birth; her physical experiences and interactions with her environment are all part of what inform her developing brain and body.

concerned about the movement stages being difficult for that baby; I'm also concerned about them creating habits of SNS arousal. That is to say, the hindbrain is learning the state of arousal as the predominant state, and the baby has a good chance of being in constant low-grade arousal throughout childhood and into adulthood. Remember that baby's system is very immature at birth; her physical experiences and interactions with her environment are all part of what inform her developing brain and body.

There are many reasons a baby may be in extension/arousal mode more often than flexion/calm mode. Again, let's not assume all extension is bad and to be avoided. For example, babies use extension to communicate frustration by stiffening and arching their backs. But again, we want babies to move freely with a balance of flexion and extension and not be stuck in or leading from either state.

A great example of how babies first experience the balance of flexion and extension in their physical *and* emotional development is through a primitive reflex, the Moro reflex. If you've ever seen a baby startle at a loud noise, you've witnessed the Moro reflex in action. The baby quickly extends her limbs and calls for help with a loud cry. A responsive mom or dad comes, folds her limbs back toward the center of her body, and soothes her. The job of the Moro reflex is to summon help when there is a perceived threat. There are two distinct actions in this reflex: extension and flexion. In order for this reflex to properly mature and ensure baby doesn't get stuck in extension (thus increasing the chance her body will create patterns of SNS arousal), it is crucial that baby also completes the reflex each time by flexing in, thus finding a feeling of calm by activating the PNS. The baby cannot always fold herself back up to activate her PNS; an adult is necessary to complete this action. This is one way we teach babies to self-soothe. By helping baby find a feeling of safety and calm, she will be able to find it on her own later in life. I think we all know older children and even adults who are in a constant pursuit to find something to calm them. Please give your baby the gift of feeling this sense of safety deep in her body so it becomes part of her and she won't need to seek it out so aggressively as she matures. She will just know it, because you showed her.

Helping Babies Find Their Calm

Now, back to those things that can cause baby to be in arousal more often than is optimal, thus instilling habits of imbalance in her social-emotional regulation. Your baby's nervous system responds to perceived threats. She perceives these threats through her body. Babies can perceive things as threats that we adults would not, because we have much more experience in the world and fully developed brains. Some of the things that frighten babies we can control; some we cannot. More important than protecting your baby from every possible perceived threat is to calm her and help her self-regulate and find balance and recuperation when scary or frustrating things occur. (We will talk about ways to do that later in this chapter.) Babies may feel threatened by cold, hunger, being far away from Mom and Dad, loud noises, quick changes in body position or of light in a room, unpleasant tactile experiences like tickling, or an especially difficult delivery. As you can see, common threats can sometimes be avoided, but not always.

During birth and the early days of a baby's life, she is getting a picture of what the world is like through her body and its senses; we often call this an imprint. When a baby perceives a threat during pregnancy or delivery, it becomes part of her imprint, her picture of the world. This explains why some babies seem to be in SNS arousal from day one, even though the adults have done everything right by keeping baby safe, warm, and loved. I cannot stress enough that what a baby perceives as a threat may not really be life threatening. But all that matters is her perception, and an immature system experiences threats much more readily than ours do; it also does not have our ability to rationalize a situation. If you sense your baby might need some support to self-soothe and invite the PNS, rest at ease—there are simple things you can do to help your baby find her calm and balance.

Signs Your Baby May Need Extra Support Finding Her Calm

- You feel in your heart he needs some support, which is always the best measure—please trust your inner wisdom
- She arches back and fusses a lot. (Most babies do this to communicate, but you may feel your baby does it more frequently than is typical.)
- He's very fussy and inconsolable
- Her legs and arms feel stiff and straight, not easy to bend and fold in.
- He's very uncomfortable with tummy time
- She does not like cuddling or being close and soft with you
- He only wants to be held. (This is normal for newborns, but if your older baby doesn't enjoy time on his own playing on the floor, he might need support finding his calm.)

How to Support Baby in Finding His Calm

A calm and safe baby is not only primed for healthy emotional development, but is also better able to grow the higher parts of the brain. A well-developed hindbrain, including a sense of safety and knowing that his needs will be met, will actually trigger the development of the higher parts of the brain. When baby perceives the world is safe, he can use his resources for language development and higher-order thinking skills. When baby does not have this feeling of safety, the development of the midbrain and cortex may be compromised. Below are six suggestions for helping your baby find his calm.

Take Advantage of Feeding Time

Feeding time can be a great opportunity to invite calm. First, find a quiet room to feed your baby, ideally one with dim lights. If you have older children, you may want to get them started with a quiet activity before feeding—remember, this is baby's special time. While feeding your baby, make sure to keep his arms and legs folded in and to hold him gently but firmly. Whether you are breastfeeding or bottle-feeding, this closeness and warmth paired with physical nourishment sends a powerful message to your baby about safety and getting his needs met.

Allow for Freedom of Movement

Keeping baby in devices that restrict movement compromises the optimal development of physical, emotional, and cognitive development. Babies need to feel safe in their body and that starts by being allowed to explore it in a natural way. Devices that hold up baby drastically reduce the level of intimacy a baby can have with gravity, and hence her own body and its limitations. When baby grows to know and fully understand her body in relationship to all planes, she has developed her body and a safe and calm place to be. This will serve her for her whole life.

Apply Gentle and Firm Compression on the Joints

Firm, gentle pressure to the hips and shoulders can be very soothing for baby. It will also assist him in finding his inner sense of peace and calm. Gently press on baby's knees or feet in the direction of his hip sockets. Press slowly and watch baby's face: if he shows signs of distress, ease up or try another time. I like to say in a singsong voice, "Here's Matthew," while I'm pressing down and gazing into baby's eyes. This helps baby feel a deep sense of his center and also gives him satisfying feedback about where his body is.

Attend to Your Baby When She Is Upset

Your baby must feel sure that when she needs you, you will be there. This is how she determines that she is in a safe world where her needs will be met. Your baby is not mature or sophisticated enough to manipulate you, nor is she savvy enough to cry wolf. When your baby cries, she needs you, period. A need for food or a diaper change is just as valid and deserving of attention as her need to be close to you or to be held.

There will of course be times when you can't rush to your baby's side. In these cases, you can use your soothing voice to reassure her that you hear her and she is safe. When baby is a bit older, you can simply say, "Mommy's hands are busy, but I'm close." You may also want to have a song or two you can sing to baby when you can't pick her up. Again, as babies grow, the methods we use to attend to them can expand as well. But please, always attend.

Honor Your Baby's Signs

If your baby seems scared of a family member wishing to hold him or is just not in the mood to be passed around, honor that by keeping him close and using a firm, loving hold while rocking and soothing him. Understandably, this can be tricky to navigate with loved ones at first, but it won't last. You may just say to the other person, "Let's let him get adjusted for a few minutes, then we can try again." You can also continue to talk with the other adult and let baby be part of the conversation while he's in your arms. It's common for adults to be so excited to see baby and this excitement may be scary for baby. When I greet parents in my office or even out and about at the store, I spend time connecting with Mom or Dad by talking to them and making eye contact, hugging them when appropriate, helping with their diaper bag, etc.

Baby will sense I am a safe person when she senses that Mom and Dad are at ease with me. Then I very gently direct my attention to the baby when it feels right. When excited loved ones approach baby, try using a very quiet voice with them and engage them in conversation to set the mood before directing the attention to baby.

Protect Your Baby from Overpowering Stimuli

As adults, we enjoy a certain amount of stimulus. We might watch exciting television shows or listen to loud music. We might stay out late, go to brightly lit amusement parks, hang out in crowded mall, or watch fireworks. The adult nervous system can withstand this kind of stimulus, because we have fully developed brains that allow us to process what is happening. The infant brain is different. It requires far less stimulus than the adult brain to grow. In fact, too much stimulus is actually harmful to a developing baby's brain.

> too much stimulus is actually harmful to a developing baby's brain.

We know that when the hindbrain is allowed to develop naturally, it stimulates the cortex, which leads to higher brain functioning. We also know that baby has to feel safe for the higher parts of the brain to develop. Finally, we know that inappropriate sensory stimuli will trigger a baby into perceiving a threat. So, if we want our baby's hindbrain to be healthy, we need to limit the sensory stimuli around it. This includes bright lights, loud noises, televisions, and computers.

> child development research clearly indicates that love, touch, cuddling, and soothing your baby are more important than anything you can buy.

Parents, particularly new ones, can feel pressure to buy their babies all the latest toys and gadgets, anything to give them a "leg up" on learning. What I find so curious is that while this over-stimulating approach emphasizes the number of books or special toys in a house, or trying to teach your children as much as possible before they start school, child development research clearly indicates that love, touch, cuddling, and soothing your baby are more important than anything you can buy.

Wear Baby When You're Running Errands

Related to the last point: I understand that we all must bring baby to run errands from time to time. When you do, consider wearing baby in a carrier close to you and keeping a light blanket over his head. The lights and action inside the local department store are too much for a baby; this is the kind of place he will certainly need help finding his calm, so do all you can to assist him. For example, when my son was young, car rides were hard for him. To give him a settling moment while running errands, I used to nurse him in the car in store parking lots before driving to the next place.

If your baby is quiet in these places, that does not mean he isn't overly stimulated. When stimulation overwhelms an immature system, the system will often protect itself by shutting out the stimulus. So continue doing all you can to soothe your baby in high-stimulus environments, even when he appears calm.

Care for Your Own Nervous System

As a busy mother, I know all too well how difficult this is. After a long day with many demands on my time, energy, and patience, it can be extremely challenging to remember how important it is to care for myself. But self-care is crucial, not just for me but for my son. This goes beyond self-help talk or Oprah-inspired messages. Your baby's brain development, in part, relies on your self-care. Remember your baby picks up on your inner state and feels the level of stress in your body. Your supported, calm nervous system communicates to your baby that the world is safe.

In addition to feeling your soft, calm body, another way your baby learns from you is through mirror neurons. These neurons fire exactly the same way in the brain when a person does an action or watches an action. For example, if I watch someone kick a ball, the same neurons fire as if I was physically kicking the ball myself. Think of the implications this has when teaching your baby how to be in the world. If we want them to take care of themselves someday, the most powerful way to teach them is to do the same.

A healthy, calm, and balanced parent is the best teacher for a child. This means that you are eating nourishing food and drinking plenty of water, which will give you strength to care for your baby. It means you are getting moderate exercise and respecting your body's needs. It means you are taking breaks for self-care, even if it's just thirty minutes to shower and eat. It means you are getting enough rest.

New parents may read this and laugh, and I understand that impulse. In addition to having to balance the demands of life, we Americans live in increasingly isolated family units of one or two parents and children. Throughout human history, support systems have included extended families, villages, or tribes in which adults, most often women, shared responsibility for raising children. In today's world, these traditional practices are fading fast or gone completely, for better or worse. Even so, I urge you to find a support system for yourself, for your well-being and your child's. Try a parenting group or a new parent club, or reach out to your parents, grandparents, or friends. Don't be afraid to ask for help. Remember that your emotional and physical balance is as important for your child as it is for you.

Talk in Simple, Declarative Statements

An infant brain is a kind of sponge, absorbing all stimuli around it. Your baby is looking to you for information on how to respond to and handle our complicated world. By speaking to your baby in simple, reassuring statements, you are offering her a banquet of language. For example, say it's lunchtime. A loving and playful parent might be tempted to ask in a high-pitched and excited voice, "Are you hungry? Should we eat something? What's this? Do you remember what this is?" This kind of questioning creates stress in a growing mind. Instead, consider calmly stating, "It's lunch time. Let's see what we have. Oh look, we have a banana. You like bananas. They are yellow and sweet." You can also eat with your baby and continue the conversation with: "Mmm, this is delicious. All right, now your turn. Open up," and so on. While we want to offer baby plenty of exposure to words, we want practice using language that is not in the form of a question. This is harder than it may seem! When my son was a baby, we had a jar on the kitchen table and put a dime in it each time a question was asked to a little baby with limited language to help us break the habit!

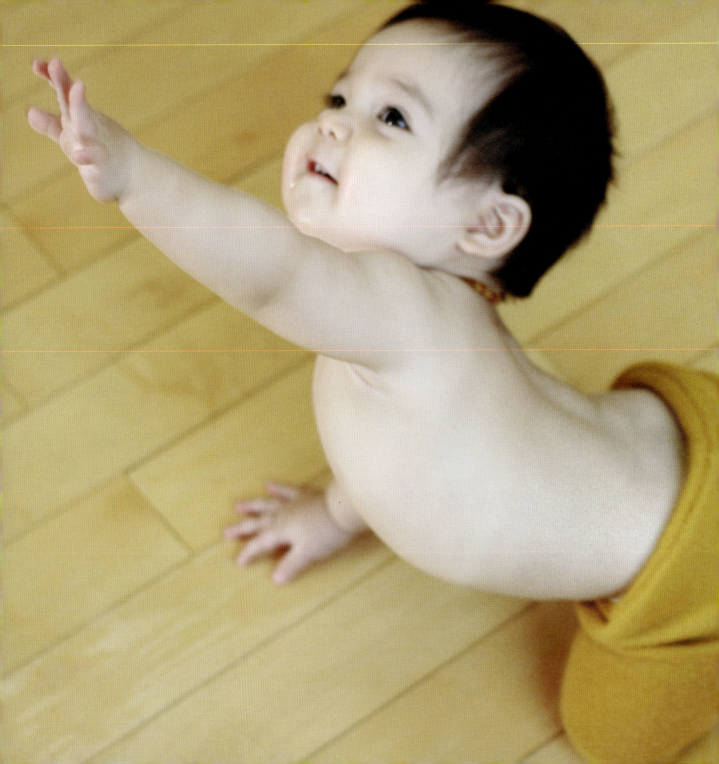

5

Hemisphere Integration

As humans, our distinct advantage over other creatures is the size and power of our brains. In fact, the human brain is so powerful and sophisticated that during the course of human development, it divided into two different hemispheres, or halves. This separation allowed each hemisphere to specialize in specific functions. When working together, they become even stronger.

Let's look at the two hemispheres a little more closely.

- **Right hemisphere:** The right side of our brain helps us see the whole picture and focus on the big idea. It sees things in images and textures and considers ideas broadly. While reading, the right hemisphere sees an entire word, like *dinosaur*.
- **Left hemisphere:** The left side of our brain breaks things into smaller, doable chunks. It focuses on language and details. It analyzes and decodes symbols. While reading, the left hemisphere breaks a word down into pieces, like *die-no-sawr*.

To function at our best, we need both halves of our brains working together, or integrated. When our two hemispheres are integrated and talk to each other, we can do things like read, solve problems, play sports, and tackle math and science.

Some of us may identify with one side of our brains more than the other. For instance, an artist might think he is more "right brained" while a scientist might think she is more "left brained." In reality, we all use both sides of our brains every day. It's true that we all have a hemisphere dominance that leads when we are confronted with a novel situation or problem; however, it is optimal to use them both as a team. But how do the two hemispheres work together?

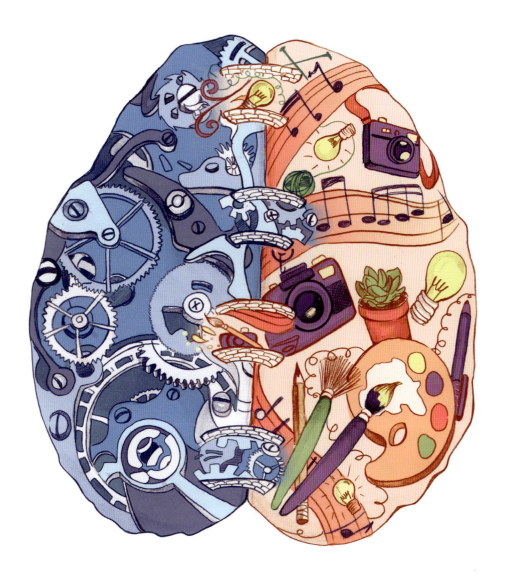

The ability to access both hemispheres is directly linked to early movement patterns. The more your baby moves freely as an infant, the stronger the bridges between right and left hemispheres will be.

Hemisphere Integration

> When our two hemispheres are integrated and talk to each other, we can do things like read, solve problems, play sports, and tackle math and science.

The Bridge between the Hemispheres

One of the parts of the brain that helps the two hemispheres work as a team is the corpus callosum. The corpus callosum is a bundle of fibers that acts like a bridge between the right and left halves, sending messages back and forth inside our brain. An ideal corpus callosum is a fat bundle of fibers that transmits information quickly between the right and left hemispheres.

So, as a parent, how can you help your child build a big, strong corpus callosum? For one, you can allow and encourage crosslateral movement. That is, by supporting your child through his innate developmental movement stages, he will naturally arrive at crosslateral movement when he creeps on all fours. This crosslateral movement works both sides of the brain, helping the two hemispheres integrate. This integration, this communication between the hemispheres, will be crucial later in life. It's like going to the gym and using free weights to strengthen opposing muscle groups. Only instead of building strong arms or legs, your baby is using crosslateral movement to build a strong bridge between hemispheres.

When a child has a robust corpus callosum and well-integrated brain hemispheres, she will be able to do all sorts of things. She will be able to perform physical tasks like running, skipping, and throwing a ball with grace and ease. When she gets older, she will also be able to perform complex intellectual tasks. An important example of this is the ability to apply known facts to novel situations. Picture a child who can recite multiplication tables perfectly. When she gets older, she will encounter story problems in math class

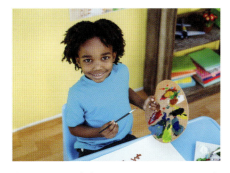 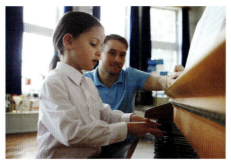

Creating art and playing an instrument require the use of both hemispheres.

("John has three dollars and wants to buy gum that costs twenty-five cents per piece. How many pieces of gum can he buy?"). If this girl who knows her times tables has a strong corpus callosum and integrated hemispheres, this problem will be easier for her. She will be able to apply her known facts (the multiplication tables) to this novel situation.

Parents will also see evidence of this ability in their children's everyday lives. If you have an older child, you may have instilled certain routines in his home life. For example, maybe before going to bed he first gets into pajamas, then brushes his teeth, and finally reads a story. But when he goes to Grandma's, he may have difficulty translating his routine to this novel situation. As another example, you may have taught your child at home that when he walks in the door, he should take off his shoes and hang up his coat. But when he first goes to school, he may have a hard time applying this routine to his new surroundings. A strong, integrated brain will help him make these kinds of transitions more smoothly.

Hemisphere Integration and Reading

The old saying is still true: "Reading is fundamental." Reading is absolutely necessary for success in our society, from reading the news to stay informed to reading instructions on tax forms or job applications. And for school-aged children, reading is not only necessary in English class but is also one of the primary methods for learning other subjects like biology or history. How many of us remember lugging around science or social studies textbooks filled with words we'd need to understand? Reading is the basis for learning in school, and without solid reading skills, a student will slip farther and farther behind his peers.

The bottom-up approach to child development will help your child read. Period. By reading this sentence, you are demonstrating that the hemispheres of your brain are integrated. Your eyes are moving across the page smoothly on their own as you take in this information. You don't have to consciously force them to move smoothly. Think of how tiring it would be if you had to focus on moving your eyes to read. It would take so much work you wouldn't process the information as easily. For comparison, think about how easy it is to walk across a room. You simply stand and move. Now imagine how hard it would be if you had to consciously think about moving each foot as you walked. All of your energy would go toward the simple act of walking. The same is true of reading.

Part of what makes reading and walking feel effortless is the ability to cross the midline of the body. It's easy to see how we do that while walking, but we also do it while reading. Think of the eyes tracking from one side of the page to the other; at some point, those eyes have to cross the middle of the body at the bridge of the nose to get to the other side. When that occurs effortlessly and seamlessly, we can read with ease. When hemispheres are not well integrated, instead of the eyes tracking smoothly, they skip at the midline and this can cause complications with reading, including:

- Trouble keeping your place
- Poor comprehension skills
- Slow pace

- Reading below grade level
- Symptoms of dyslexia

Our goal is to build the mechanics of reading in a child's brain early on so that when it is time to start reading, the cortex is free to handle the tasks of decoding symbols, sounding out words, making meaning, and visualizing what is being read. When we use movement to nurture strong hemisphere integration in our children's brains early in life, we help ensure that they have those mechanics.

The human body is a mirror for how the brain is working. In my own clinical practice, I have seen a direct link between how a child moves and the difficulties she experiences in school. Those difficulties are, in part, due to a lack of unrestricted movement opportunities early in life.

Summary

- Over many years, human brains developed specialized halves called hemispheres, each with its own strengths.
- The corpus callosum acts as the bridge between them, helping them to integrate, or work together.
- A strong corpus callosum will enable a child to do well in school and beyond.
- You can help your child build a strong corpus callosum, and an integrated brain, by allowing freedom of movement during infancy that will result in the ability to do crosslateral movement.

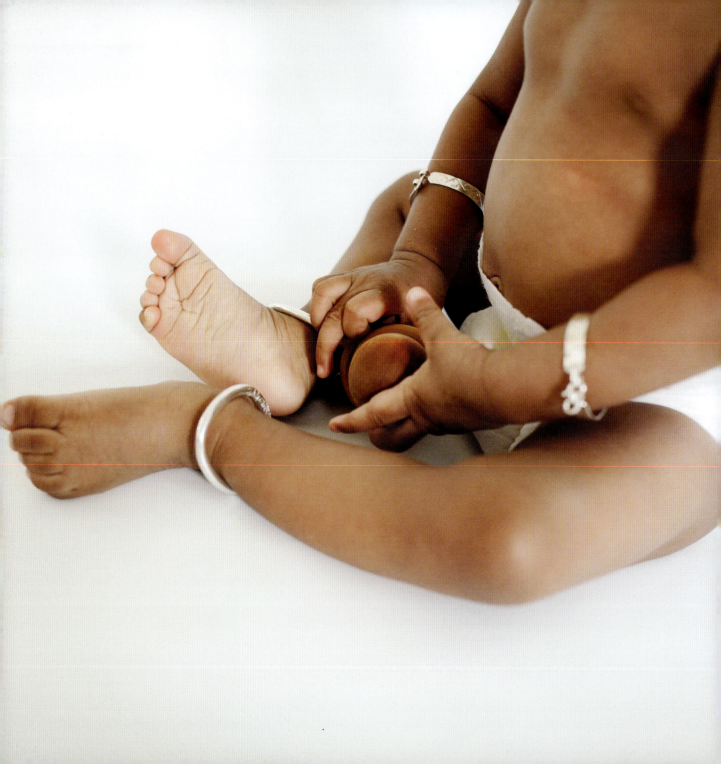

6

Our Wonderful Inner Senses

When we hear the word *senses*, we automatically think of those five senses we were taught when we were kids—sight, smell, taste, touch, and hearing. In addition to these important outer senses, we are actually born with something called inner senses.

So far, we have talked about how your baby will build his brain through bodily movement. He will also build his brain through his inner and outer senses, which are also part of the nervous system and closely linked with early movement and brain development.

While we have many inner senses that work alongside the outer senses, in this book we will investigate only a few. First, let's take a closer look at two crucial inner senses: the **vestibular** and **proprioceptive senses.**

The Vestibular Sense

Your vestibular system includes the semicircular canals of the inner ear, the cerebellum, the core muscles of the body, and even the eyes. It is the first system in the human body to develop; in fact, the vestibular system is fully developed in utero by the time a fetus is sixteen weeks old. The fact that the vestibular system develops so early indicates how important it is for human growth, and thus how important movement is to all future development.

The vestibular system tells your brain where your body is in space. In a nutshell, the vestibular sense is the ability to know where you are in relation to the center of the earth. Your vestibular sense regulates your sense of balance, guides your sense of direction, and helps you understand where you are in relationship to things you see and hear. Think of using a level to make sure a picture is hanging straight. You know the picture is balanced when the fluid inside the level is centered. Your vestibular system acts like a level inside your inner ear. But what does this mean for babies?

Since your baby's vestibular system fully develops while she is still in utero, she already has a sense of orientation within the aquatic world of your womb before she is even born. After birth, she will continue to develop her vestibular system to master important life skills. And the way to build a strong vestibular system is, you've probably guessed, through movement—once again, movement directly builds the brain!

Here are some skills that rely on the vestibular sense:

- Overall balance
- Postural and motor skills like head control, sitting, and walking
- Developing appropriate muscle tone
- Overall energy
- Sense of direction
- Spatial perception
- Ability to sit still
- Body coordination
- Spatial problem-solving
- Organizational skills
- Maintaining appropriate personal space with others
- Writing

When you physically know the direction of your own body in space (down, up, left, right), you can make appropriate shapes on a page, which is essential for writing, and recognize shapes, which is essential for reading. If your body is confused about where it is in space, it is very difficult to draw a vertical line with a bubble on the lower right-hand side, as in the letter *b*. So many learning and attention challenges can be traced to a poorly developed vestibular system.

How can you help your baby develop her vestibular sense? You can feed her from both sides. You can rock her gently. You can use a wrap that allows you to wear her throughout the day. That way, when you experience the world, she will experience it with you. When you bend forward, she will bend forward, and when you reach for something, she will see how far away from you it is. This will help her understand where she is in space. Anything that keeps your baby close to you, allowing her to feel your movements in space, will help.

Freedom to move on her own will also develop baby's vestibular sense. Remember in the roly-poly stage, when baby rolls from front to back for the first time? That is a big moment in the process of developing the vestibular sense. In one swift motion, baby's body orientation and view totally shifts. If a baby is confined and not allowed to explore different places and spatial relationships, the development of her vestibular system will be compromised, which may cause problems later in life. So baby holders that confine her movements can inhibit the development of her vestibular sense. This is why keeping her close to you (where she can feel your body in space) or on the floor (where she is free to move) is ideal.

Allow your baby to explore gravity and her body in gravity. Remember to avoid sitting her up before she is ready. The journey to sitting is huge for the development of the inner senses; placing baby in a foam baby chair or helping her sit in any way only robs her of the chance to develop these crucial inner senses. Through freedom of movement, she will better understand where she is as an entity separate from the things around her. She will then feel more confidence as she explores future stages.

The Proprioceptive Sense

While the vestibular sense is the awareness of where your body is in relation to the center of the earth, proprioception is the awareness of where your body parts are in relation to other body parts. Proprioception also tells you where your body ends and someone else's body begins. It is the internal sense of the physical self that enables us to complete detailed maneuvers without conscious awareness and in the absence of other sensory clues. Proprioceptors are located throughout the body in the joints, tendons, and muscles, enabling us to make minute adjustments for fine muscle coordination based on direct sensory input.

Close your eyes and touch the tip of your nose with your right index finger—you just used your proprioception. You were able to figure out where your nose was in relation to your arm. If your proprioception was underdeveloped for some reason, you may have missed your nose by overshooting it or not reaching far enough.

What does this mean for babies? Proprioception helps your baby understand the physical boundaries of her body. Very early on, your baby uses her proprioception to understand where her body ends and her mother's begins. Many educators, neuroscientists, and clinicians believe that proprioception is the first language. That is, if we think of language as communication, then proprioception allows us to receive and give communication through our bodies. When baby is lying on her back, her parent might gently press on her foot. In response, baby will press back. This is a form of communication. It tells the parent her signal was received and mirrors that signal back to her. This kind of give and take creates a blueprint for attunement later in life. It helps develop your baby's ability to receive communication and body input and respond appropriately.

When my son, August, was a baby I remember gently squeezing his hips and shoulders to help calm him when he was agitated. When a baby gets this deep feedback about where his body is, it sends a soothing and reassuring feeling throughout the body; this can be one of the first ways we teach self-regulation. With clients of all ages who experience overstimulation, anxiety, or restlessness, I apply similar gentle but deep compression to the hips and shoulders while saying, "Here's Jordon" or "Here's Natalie," the same way I did with August when he was a baby. I watch their bodies find center and their faces become focused. Their energy becomes grounded in their bodies rather than scattering all over the room.

I see many children in my practice who struggle with proprioceptive development. With well-developed proprioception your baby will be less likely to experience the following symptoms as he grows older:

- Poor posture
- Clumsiness
- Constant fidgeting, even while sitting still
- Falling or tossing body against walls (to receive feedback about his body)
- Tendency to press or push against others (again, to receive sensory feedback)
- Poor understanding of personal space
- Excessive desire to be held
- Visual problems

To help develop proprioception, you can give your baby deep, gentle squeezes all over his body. While he is lying in front of you on his back, you can push firmly against the bottom of his foot. When he feels this, he may push back. This silent conversation between parent and baby helps baby understand that his body has boundaries, and that sensory input from outside his body relates to actions from inside his body.

Hearing, Sight, and Brain Development

Inspired in part by revelations about severe neglect in Romanian orphans in the sixties, U.S. researchers became interested in the effects of institutionalization on children in subsequent decades. Numerous studies have shown that children who are completely deprived of stimulation demonstrate more difficulty in forming attachments and lower brain activity than their non-institutionalized peers.

With the very best intentions, American mainstream culture swung to the opposite end of the spectrum: overstimulation. We created toys, games, books, electronic devices, television shows, videos, and music all designed to encourage our children's growing minds. But what we ended up creating was a world with entirely too much stimulation, flooded by a cacophony of sounds and blinking lights; television shows that jump back and forth between scenes faster than the brain can follow; and toys that beep and flash in response to the slightest touch. In the face of all this overpowering stimulation, what happens to a fragile, developing brain?

A constant barrage of sound early in life can discourage babies, and later children, from developing true listening skills. When confronted with nonstop noise, a baby's nervous system will want to shut down to protect itself. She will shut out or ignore certain sounds from an early age. She will not develop the ability to analyze and distinguish sounds on a minute level, which could adversely affect her speech and reading. Even if her speech develops at an appropriate age, those minute distinctions in sound could be lost on her. She may not be able to hear the difference between similar or blended sounds, such as *ch* and *sh* or *p* and *b*. This inability to hear the differences could affect her ability to read and write.

Every parent wants to help her baby develop a strong, powerful brain. The good news is that you don't need fancy, expensive toys or games to do this. The simplest, most basic sounds are enough for your baby's fragile brain. Muted balls, wooden shakers, the seedpods that fall from catalpa trees—all of these soft sounds provide ample stimulation for any baby. But perhaps the most interesting and stimulating sound for your baby is the sound of your voice. When you talk, sing, or hum to your baby, the vibrations from your vocal chords resonate with your baby's vocal chords, and that helps her learn how to speak. This resonance does not occur when listening to television or the radio. In fact, the language on television and radio is very fast and devoid of any natural pauses. It is hard to distinguish separate words and hear the natural rhythm of language. It is also digitized, and therefore missing a lot of the overtones and harmonics that exist in the human voice and in analog sound (like on old records). With most digital recordings we lose some of the sound spectrum.

Similarly, anything found in nature will both fascinate your baby and help her brain develop beautifully. You do not need to give her brightly colored toys with flashing lights; simple toys made of natural fibers like wood, silk, and wool are perfect toys for your baby. The simple gradations of color found in a field of grass or on a tree trunk are enough to stimulate her brain. In humans, the visual processing center of the brain and the eyes are not fully integrated until prepuberty. By providing an environment that encourages your child to see minute variations in color, texture, and shape found in the three-dimensional world, you help build that connection between her brain and eyes.

. . . .

With good intentions, we have gotten in the habit of overstimulating babies and children. The size and amount of stimulus should mirror the size of the child; stimulus that is too big can compromise the sensory development of a baby. The world is so new to babies that they do not need the level of stimulus adults have become accustomed to in order to be entertained. Even small, simple objects can pique their curiosity and hold their attention.

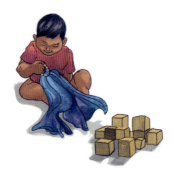

It's All about Proportion

Another way to look at overstimulation of your baby is to consider the size, fragility, and immaturity of their system as compared to the stimulus—ideally they should be proportionate. For example, you wouldn't give your newborn a five-course meal, but a loud toy that blinks and shakes when touched is just as inappropriate for your baby's fragile sensory system as a meal of steak and potatoes are for his digestion. When you watch your baby coo and squirm you can tune in to how delicate he really is, find toys and expose him only to those things that are soft and manageable for him. A wooden rattle with a soft muted sound or a colorful silk for a gentle game of peek-a-boo pair perfectly with baby. When sights and sounds are too big for baby, she must protect herself by either turning off and tuning out, or bracing and shrieking and making herself bigger and louder to match the stimulus. The ideal environments for baby are those that he does not need to retreat from or brace against, those that meet baby right where he is—that is when baby is able to truly engage with something and explore it. Think about your delicate new baby versus a big-screen television. He is no match for that. The screen and its images and sound are not in proportion to your baby—they are entirely too big. This is again why nature provides such a perfect play environment for young children: leaves, light rain, a breeze, sticks, and a bird's chirping are all just the right amount of stimulus for baby. Inside the house, soft singing of your voice or soft music, natural light streaming in the window, simple toys made of natural materials and don't require batteries, and the sounds of meal preparation in the kitchen are all in proportion to your baby and are enough to stimulate his senses.

Summary

- While there are many inner and outer senses, the vestibular sense and proprioception are truly crucial to optimal brain development and closely connected to movement.
- Both are key to the development of other senses as well as the nervous system.
- If either of these senses doesn't fully develop, it could contribute to many problems for children later in life.
- Hearing and sight are two crucial outer senses that are also inextricably linked to brain development and movement.
- As parents, the best way to help our children develop is to protect them from too much sensory stimulation and instead provide an environment full of gentle sounds and sights that are optimal for infant development.

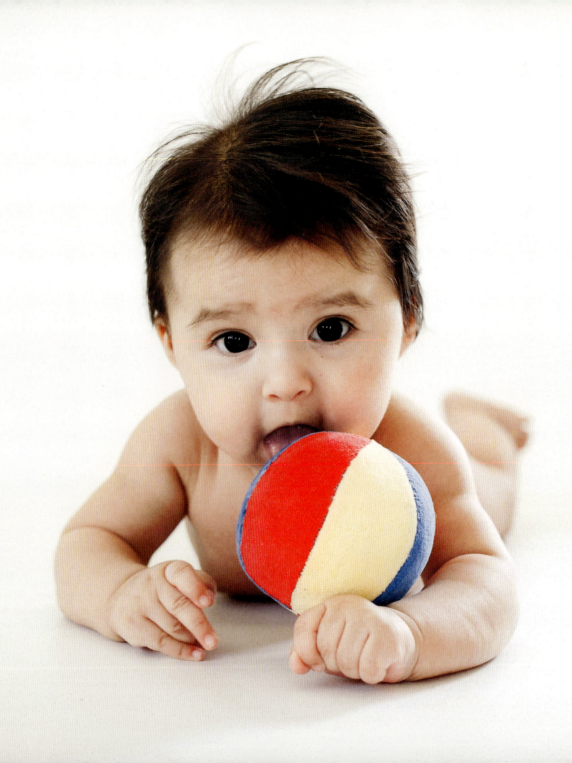

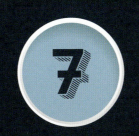

What's Getting in the Way of Healthy Brain Development?

Throughout this book, we've learned how a bottom-up approach to child development builds strong brains. We've also learned that healthy brain development results from allowing children to move freely through their innate developmental stages with a feeling of safety. It is not an exaggeration to say that the rest of your child's life is dependent on what happens during that window of birth to eighteen months. How he learns, how he manages emotional and social situations, how well he does in school, and how he functions in society depend on whether or not he was able to fully develop his hindbrain during this window.

If building a strong, integrated brain is so natural, why do so many American children seem to have such a hard time in school? The National Assessment of Education Progress reports that 66 percent of American fourth graders cannot read at grade level, with an even more concerning 80 percent of fourth graders from low-income families performing under grade level. The Anxiety and Depression Association of America states that one in eight children has anxiety, and the CDC states that 11 percent of children between the ages of four and seventeen have ADD/HD—that is 6.4 million children in 2011, with evidence the number is rising. What's getting in the way of healthy brain development? While there are *many* factors involved in this crisis that go beyond the scope of this book, we will address only those factors related to movement and brain development. In this chapter, we'll consider some of the ways we—as parents, adults, educators, or Americans—might be unconsciously inhibiting our children's brain development.

What's Polluting the Oak Tree?

As parents we want to give our children as much as we can. And we happen to live in a culture in which we think more is more. That is, we are constantly told that if we buy this or that product for our child, he will be better off. But the reality is that less is more. As I've said from the beginning of this book, your child was born with all the tools he needs within his body and brain to grow into a smart, successful, loved, and loving human being. This takes time—there is no value to rushing this process.

Remember that tall oak tree we talked about in the first chapter? We want to give an oak tree everything it needs to grow. We want to make sure it gets lots of sunlight and rain, with plenty of room for its roots and branches to spread out. We don't want to expose it to anything that might stunt its growth, like pollution or harsh chemicals, and we know that a tree like this takes time.

Like you, I want my son to grow like a giant oak tree. I want him to become strong, robust, and resilient, and I want to avoid anything that might interfere with his development. Below are a few everyday things that can get in the way of healthy brain development.

Restricted Movement

We live in a time of an unprecedented number of contraptions and gadgets to help busy parents and keep babies safe; 75 percent of babies' waking time is spent in a container of some kind. On average, babies spend six hundred hours a year in car seats alone. Car seats are necessary when driving, but how many hours does a baby spend in a car seat outside of a vehicle?

While many products claim to build better, stronger babies, they actually hinder hindbrain development by putting babies' bodies in unnatural positions for long periods. As a mother, I know timesaving devices that free up my hands can be incredibly useful. But however seductive these devices are, I also know the time a baby spends in these containers is time she is not on the floor and developing her hindbrain and body. Remember that when a baby is upright, she is using the cortex. We want the hindbrain to develop first, and that happens on the floor. The cortex has a long time to grow—scientists say it can keep growing until young adulthood and beyond! Propping baby upright

A Typical Day in the Life of an American Baby

Baby wakes up in her crib and Mom picks her up and carries her to her changing table, where she gets her diaper changed. Then Mom carries her to her high chair and feeds her breakfast. Mom carries her back to her changing table and changes her diaper again, if necessary, and dresses her. Then Mom puts baby in her car seat and carries her from the house to the car. Mom drives baby to her daycare and carries her in her car seat from the car into the daycare. The daycare provider picks baby up out of her car seat and places her in some sort of holding device. When it's time to eat, the daycare provider places baby in a high chair and feeds her. At naptime, the daycare provider places baby in a crib. At the end of the day, Mom picks up baby and places her in a car seat and carries her to the car, and then perhaps Mom drives to some errand, such as the bank. Mom places baby in car seat and carries her into the bank with her. After she is done banking, Mom carries baby in her car seat back to the car and drives baby home. Mom then carries baby in car seat into house and places her into her high chair to feed her dinner. Depending on the time, Mom may place baby into a holding container before getting ready for bed.

    Throughout her entire day, baby spends maybe twenty or thirty minutes on the floor in free movement. She spends perhaps even less time in the arms of a loving caregiver. This is happening in homes of parents all over the country who love their children and want the best for them. But, as a society, we have become misguided about what that "best" really entails. The best thing for any child is freedom of movement and a caregiver who responds to her needs—both essential for brain development.

contributes to a top-down approach by developing the cortex too early and robbing baby of crucial floor time. In addition to putting baby in a compromising position for cognitive and physical development, spending so much time in a holding container means less time in your arms feeling your touch and being close, which is also absolutely crucial for your baby's development.

Unsupported and Isolated Parents

As a busy mother, I know how hard this one can be. After working, driving through traffic, eating on the fly, and rushing through errands, it's challenging enough to get home and get food on the table, much less remember to take care of myself. But as a trained somatic psychotherapist, I need to remember that since my son was born, he's absorbed information about the world from me. Early on, my body passed on neurological messages to his. In a sense, his body acted as an extension of my nervous system. (Remember the mirror neurons that connect our behavior and actions to our baby on a deep level.) Thus, when my stress level was low and my nervous system was calm, he had a better chance of finding calm in his own body. His body received the message that "Yes, I have entered a world that is safe and where my needs will be met." When my stress level was high and my nervous system was overtaxed, he received the message that the world was not safe and his needs may not be met.

Therefore, when August was an infant, it was imperative for me to find support structures. Parents know themselves and their communities better than anyone else, so it is up to each person to figure out how best to do this. Here are a few ideas that worked for me, but you of course know what works best for you:

- Ask for help from friends or family. If you are fortunate to have family and friends that live close by, take advantage of that and

ask for help. They can hold the baby so you can shower or nap, make meals, or do some laundry, or share a cup of tea or a movie with you.
- Find a parents' group. Becoming a new parent is life changing. It is helpful to find a group of parents to connect with to share ups and downs with and just get a break from the often isolating experience of new parenthood.
- Create a babysitting co-op. Finding childcare for your infant can be hard. Who to trust? Some new parents have found that bringing together a few families that agree to take turns with each others' children can form a strong, trusted community and provide each other with support and child care for no charge.
- Seek out a spiritual community. If you find inspiration and support in a spiritual practice or community, this is a great time to reinvest in your spirituality.

One of the drawbacks of our wonderful, modern society is that we are more mobile than ever before. While traditional societies emphasized extended, multigenerational families living close to each other, oftentimes under the same roof, many parents nowadays must raise their children more or less alone. This puts added pressure on the job of parenting that, while joyful and beautiful, can also be stressful and confusing.

It is important for all of us as parents to realize that it wasn't always like this, and it's certainly not our fault that society has become this way. Most important, *know that it is vital (and okay!) to ask for help when we need it.* When you ask for help, you give someone the gift of being able to help you. Whether it's through family, friends, coworkers, or a new parent group of complete strangers, finding community to help you is crucial to your baby's healthy development.

In essence, by finding support when your baby is young, you are taking care of her so she can become a great thinker later.

Media

The American Pediatric Association recommends that children under the age of two avoid all media. In my practice, I recommend no or limited media for children until the age of eight at the very youngest, and in fact, you could extend that even further to twelve. This is difficult, since most public schools are asking young students to use media for school. The increase in media use at school means it becomes even more important that a child's leisure time is spent using their bodies, creating and exploring outdoors.

I know we live in an age of nonstop information, and that for older youth and adults, this information can be a powerful resource. But please remember that for a developing young brain, stimuli from the natural world are enough. The sound of conversation, the sight of a tree, the feel of a soft carpet, the smell of freshly cut grass or dinner being cooked, the taste of milk, a few simple toys made of natural materials—all of this is enough to feed a young child's mind. In Minneapolis and many other cities we are fortunate to have ample public green spaces all throughout the city for everyone to access. Unfortunately, not all cities and neighborhoods have enough safe green spaces for kids and parents to explore. Keeping plants in the house or finding a local community garden to participate in may be a solution for parents who do not have access to green spaces. We must all let city planners and politicians know that safe green spaces are a priority for all our children.

We know that when the hindbrain is allowed to develop naturally, it stimulates the cortex, which leads to higher brain functioning. We also know that when the sympathetic nervous system is chronically triggered, it limits hindbrain health. Finally, we know that sensory stimuli trigger the sympathetic nervous system. So if we want our baby's hindbrain to be healthy, we

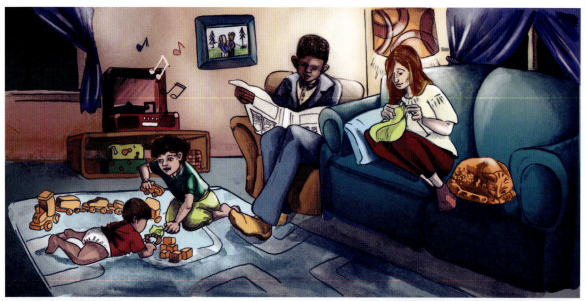
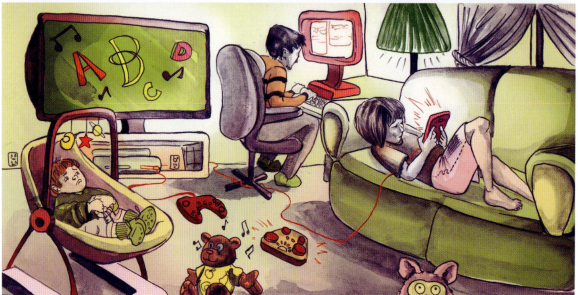

Protecting children from media and offering a movement-rich life are the two most important things you can do for your child's development.

need to limit the sensory stimuli around it. This means we try our best to limit sensory input that is too big for a baby to take in, such as flashing lights, loud noises, and too much background noise.

Media is chock full of all these things—sudden light changes, loud noises, and fast-paced music. Therefore, any moving image on a screen will trigger a baby's sympathetic arousal and hinder her brain development. It doesn't matter what the image is, whether it's a video that teaches the alphabet or plays Beethoven. All screens are detrimental to a baby's development because they hinder hindbrain growth and drastically compromise optimal development of the visual sense.

Medical Interventions

The way we are born has a great deal to do with the development of our nervous systems. While we are fortunate to have medical advances that keep mothers and babies alive and well during pregnancy and delivery, it is also true that when medical interventions are used during pregnancy and birth, the development of the nervous system is compromised.

Like many babies today, my son was delivered by caesarian section. That was not in my birth plan. I wanted an intervention-free delivery, but due to complications beyond my control, I ended up needing surgery to get him out and into my arms safely. Earlier, we learned that what a baby perceives as a threat is their reality. Although the adults supporting my birth and I all knew an operation was the safest choice, from my son's perspective, a C-section delivery and all that goes along with it was perceived as life threatening from his perspective. I found this difficult, and I lamented not having the birth I wanted. Today, at the age of seven, his nervous system continues to need support and we are working to help him feel more at ease and safe in his body and this world.

> When a child is met by nature, he knows it is safe to explore and follow his curiosities.

Regardless of the type of delivery you had with your baby, what happens after the birth can provide the nurturing and safety needed for baby to develop optimally. Proximity, warmth, unrestricted movement, music, and a supported mother all go a long way toward helping mother and baby recuperate from a tricky delivery.

Lack of Outdoor Time

Children spend less time outdoors now than ever before. Depending on how old you are, you may remember a childhood full of outdoor time where Mom and Dad would say, "Be home for dinner." For most children this is not the reality today. Our schedules are packed with activities, and most free time is spent interacting with electronic devices inside. Outdoor time offers something that indoor time cannot. Indoors is often full of things that are overly stimulating for developing nervous systems: televisions, radios, artificial light sources, electrical current coursing throughout the house. Computers and screens of all kinds fill our homes, schools, and libraries. Nature meets children where they are, moves at a pace more in line with their natural pace. The sounds of nature are just enough, the smells in nature are just enough, the sights and textures of nature are just enough. The trees, grass, birds, and rocks all reflect and mirror a child's natural state. When a child spends time outdoors, the senses get cleansed of the overly stimulating effects of our indoor lives. I often take my son to the forest to "cleanse his sensory pallet" after we have been inside too long. When a child is met by nature, he knows

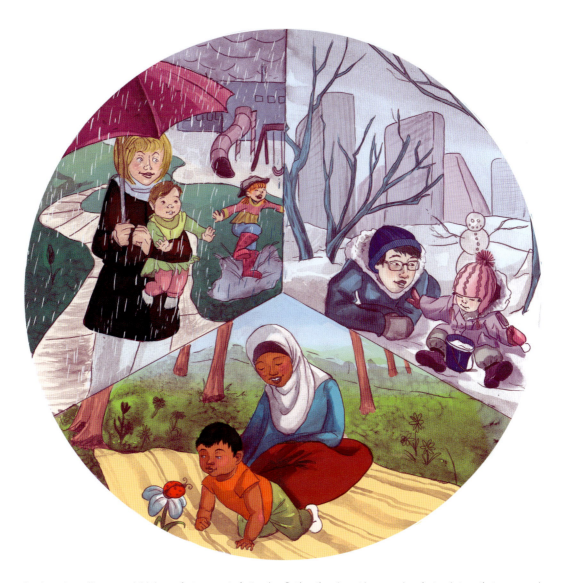

Outdoor time offers your child the perfect amount of stimulus. Rather than invest in expensive electronic toys that compromise development, I encourage you to invest in outerwear for the whole family so that you can enjoy hours of outside time in all kinds of weather.

What's Getting in the Way of Healthy Brain Development?

it is safe to explore and follow his curiosities. Spending most of our time indoors robs children of these opportunities and instead creates an environment where they are constantly bombarded by too much stimuli, which asks too much of their immature sensory systems. When faced with this, children can tire easily and have to find ways to protect themselves and/or compensate, which all compromise the optimal development of the nervous system.

In his book *The Last Child in the Woods,* Richard Louv uses the term "nature-deficit disorder" to describe the condition that occurs when children are kept from nature. As he states, "An expanding body of scientific evidence suggests that nature-deficit disorder contributes to a diminished use of the senses, attention difficulties, conditions of obesity, and higher rates of emotional and physical illnesses. Research also suggests that the nature-deficit weakens ecological literacy and stewardship of the natural world. These problems are linked more broadly to what health care experts call the 'epidemic of inactivity,' and to a devaluing of independent play. Nonetheless, we believe that society's nature-deficit disorder can be reversed."

Premature Emphasis on Academics

In an effort to raise test scores and increase overall academic achievement, Americans have been pushing academics earlier and earlier. Kindergarten used to be a year of socializing and exploring the world through stories and play. Now, even these very young children receive homework!

When my son August was five, we were outside playing in our front yard one day. We saw a neighborhood friend arriving home from school; it was about 6:00 p.m. He was just getting home from a long day of school and afterschool activities. August was of course excited to see a playmate, and he asked him to come over and play. His response was, "I can't. I have to do my homework!" As a curious child development professional, I asked, "What's your homework, buddy?" He responded, "I have to trace my letters." After a full day of academics, this five-year-old had to cut his outside play short to trace his letters? Unfortunately, this is the scenario with most children across the country.

There are countless studies that affirm that early academic pressure does not work (see resources section in back for examples). In fact, play has been found to be important to a child's physical, cognitive, and mental health by boosting problem-solving skills, risk management, language development, and independent learning skills.

Think of two twelve-year-olds, each writing an essay about an encounter with a family of frogs at a pond. One student spent most of his early years playing outside with a band of adventurers. He and his friends have actual field experience with nature for they often visit the neighborhood park, which has a forest and small pond. The other student attends a well-respected school where each child has his own laptop. This student learned about amphibians from his desk by watching an educational National Geographic program about frogs.

Whose essay do you want to read: the one by Student Nature and Friends or Student Desk and Laptop? Student Nature and Friends has actually felt warm sun on his face as he and his friends squished their toes through cold mud. He has experienced how it feels to hold a frog and see a group of tadpoles, and he has heard the sounds of the pond. Those experiences are what developed his vocabulary; he has all that real sensory information to draw on for his essay. Student Desk and Laptop has been robbed of crucial sensory experiences; in their place, he has only facts and digital images. I want to read Student Nature and Friend's essay—how about you?

The point is this: playing is not just a break from serious learning—it *is* serious learning. I'm excited to see so much research affirming the value of play. My hope is we will soon see more schools implementing early education curricula that focus on play and nature versus desks and laptops.

Summary

- Every parent, guardian, or caregiver wants to provide her child with everything the child needs to grow into a successful human being.
- We've learned in this book that babies are born with innate abilities to develop their brains naturally and at their own pace.
- As caring adults, we may be tempted to intervene with this process, but in reality, the more we invite simple, loving interactions with our babies, the more their natural process can unfold.
- One of the greatest gifts we can give our children is to create a calm and stable environment that supports their growth without too much stimulation from things like stress, sound, lights, or media.

Congratulations again on embarking on this parenting journey, and remember: *you* are all your baby needs!

(Note: If you are concerned about your baby's development beyond the suggestions made in this book, you may consider seeking hands-on support from a developmental movement therapist, somatic therapist, or biodynamic cranial sacral therapist in your area. A wonderful free online resource for further understanding why your baby may not be demonstrating the stages outlined in this book with ease and comfort can be found here: http://www.youandyourchildshealth.org/youandyourchildshealth/articles/clinic%20recommendations.html)

Glossary

Corpus Callous: a wide, flat bundle of neural fibers about 10 cm long beneath the cortex that facilitates communication between the brain hemispheres.

Crawling: mobilizing on the belly, like a lizard.

Creeping: mobilizing on hands and knees; the movement commonly referred to as "crawling" in popular culture.

Extension: the lengthening of joints in the body to straighten out limbs and spine

Flexion: the shortening of joints in the body to fold in limbs and spine

Media: for the purposes of this book: screens and devices of all kinds, including television, computers, smart phones, personal devices, video games, etc.

Parasympathetic Nervous System: The part of the autonomic nervous system that calms our body down, brings us back to calm after being upset or alerted. Often referred to as "rest and digest."

Prone: lying tummy down

Supine: lying tummy up

Sympathetic Nervous System: The part of the autonomic nervous system that activates and alerts us when danger is perceived. Commonly associated with the body's fight-or-flight responses.

References and Resources

The Dominance Profile by Carla Hannaford

Smart Moves: Why Learning Is Not All in Your Head by Carla Hannaford

Playing in the Unified Field by Carla Hannaford

From Conception to Crawling by Annie Brook

Birth's Legacy by Annie Brook

Berman, M. G., Jonides, J., & Kaplan, S. (2008). The cognitive benefits of interacting with nature. *Psychological Science, 19*, 1207–1212.

Reflexes, Behavior and Learning: A Window into a Child's Mind by Sally Goddard

The Genius of Natural Childhood Secrets of Thriving Children by Sally Goddard

What Babies and Children REALLY Need: How Mothers and Fathers Can Nurture Children's Growth for Health and Well-being by Sally Goddard Blythe

Brain Compatible Dance Education by Anne Green Gilbert

Amazing Babies by Beverly Stokes

Sensing, Feeling, and Action by Bonnie Bainbridge Cohen

Triune Brain Theory by Paul Maclean

Beyond the Rainbow Bridge: Nurturing Our Children from Birth to Seven by Barbara J. Patterson and Pamela Bradley

Endangered Minds by Jane M. Healy

The Children of Cyclops: The Influence of Television Viewing on the

Developing Human Brain by Keith Buzzell

National Scientific Council on the Developing Child (2007). *The Science of Early Childhood Development: Closing the Gap Between What We Know and What We Do.*

Moving up the Grades: Relationship between Preschool Model and Later School Success, Dr. Rebecca A Marcon, Early Childhood Research and Practice 03/2002; 4(1).

— Elizabeth Bonawitz et al., "The Double-Edged Sword of Pedagogy," *Cognition* 120 (2011): 322-30

Made Possible By:

Elke van Alen, Hamburg
Bekah Aliaghai
Rossana Alves
Anonymous
Carina and Julie Anderson
Dorothy Anderson
Jane Andrew
Aditi Angle
Andrea Atherton
Dr. Jolynn Bachman, DC
Kayla Baldwin, DC
Carrie Berlacher
Linda Bergh
Blew Family
Jessie Bollig
Mia Bolte
Rachael Bonaiuto
Mike and JoAnn Brenk
Annie Brook
Polly Brumder
Catherine Burns
Dawson-Boyd ECFE
Edwin H Caldie
Dr. Kara Carmody
Laura Cervin
Zhe Chang
Chi Gong Research Foundation
Mark Coffey
Jen Cosmano
Eve Costarelli
Marcia Cunningham
Christy Cutler
Gyula Czinano
Lori Daniels
Galen David
Lauryn M. Davin
Lisa deCathelineau
Parker Deen
Angelica DeLashmette
Laurie Delmonico
Desiree
Matthew Dornquast
Philip Doucette
Tiffany Egan
Michelle Emanuel OTR/L
Anne Estes
Lorraine Fairmont
Erica Faulkner
JoAnne Craig Ferraz
Sejal Fichadia
May Beth Fifer – SMWS
Whitney Fink
Laurie Flaherty and Rachel O'Donald, AB2 LLC
Pam Formosa, Occupational Therapist/ Developmental Specialist
Jessie Forston
Sierra Armién Funk
Lori Gallardo
Megan Gangl
Alex Gatsis
Anne G. Gilbert
Maggie Gilbert
Beth Giles
Lindsay Grabb
Elizabeth Grambusch
Jean Grech
Jennifer Guiney
Brenda Haak
Kendall Hagensen
Carole Hanlein
Harpole Family
Michelle Hartney
Health Foundations Birth Center and Amy Johnson-Grass
Naomi J. Heitz
Nicole Hendrickson
Chelsey Henney, DC
Mandy Herrick
John Hoffman
Shad Holland
Karma Hughes
Queen JEM
Jessica A Jobaris
Alexis Johnson and Melinda Garry
Graham Johnson
Karen D. Johnson
Mike Johnson
Wendy Johnson
Nancy Joy
Mariane Judd
Tom Kanthak
Jamie A Ryan Karels
Shannon Kennedy
Kindermusik of the Valley
Lacie Kmetz
Lori Kochevar
Nate Kokernot
Anne and Dominik Kulakowski
Kullman Family
Tate Leyba
London Waldorf School
Krista Lucas
Kristefor, Erin, and Ruby Lysne
Amanda Blair MacDonald
Melissa Mailly
Katie Dutch Martin
Martha Mathis
Kevin McCarthy
Kathleen McCartin
Leslie McCormick
Megan McCready
Vanessa J. B. McGuire
Hope Ann McKinzie
Eileen McMonigal
Jean Miller
Monty Miller
Lekha Krishna Minnaganti
Michael Minney
Glenda Monasch, Therapeutic Eurythmist
Dr. Amber Moravec
Kacey Morrow
Andrea Mueller
Becca Ó Murchadha
Erin Niedermaier
James Oliver
Stephanie Ortmeier
Joann N. Parker
Anthony Parr
Rosa Pasarin
Andrew Paulson
Pam Paulson
Kristina Perkins
Verita Perry
Bill Pine
Dr. Keith Prussing
Elyce Perico
Kathleen Porter
Amy Quale
Radiance Bellavita
Dr. Veronika Rákli
Diana Razumny
Kim Rector
Patricia Rendon
Anna Ritter
Lynn Rozen
Victoria Ruiz
Sally
Conradine Sanborn
Dorothy Sauser-Monnig
Emily Savage
Richard A. Schutta
Dave Schwier
Margaret Scott
Erica Sigal
Allyson Sipple
Julie Stauffer
Marcy Stempler
Doreen Stockman
Francesca Todesco
Sarah M. Tran
Jeanne Traxler and Robert Goisman
Cobus & Carike du Toit
Grace Veker
E Websper
Gideon Weick
Zachary Welch
Ashley Welz
Audrey Wiebe
Willow and Sprout
Margaret Wise
Maria Ann Youngs

Sponsors:

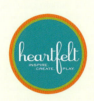

Heartfelt, owned by Lisa MacMartin, offers creative birthday parties, drop-in crafts, art and craft supplies, and natural gifts and toys. An eclectic mix of local artisan goods make unique gifts. Drop in to make one of our craft projects (they change monthly) or just come hang out in one of our comfy chairs to feel the relaxed vibe. Fairy houses are a specialty!

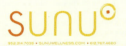

SuNu's team works to collaborate with our clients, nurture them, and customize their wellness plans using chiropractic, nutrition, acupuncture, massage, and mental health services. Our vision, training, and welcoming environment make us the preferred place for prenatal, postnatal, and pediatric care.

About the Author:

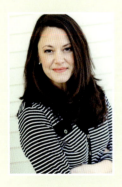

Stephanie Johnson, MA, R-DMT, LPC, is a mother, educator, registered dance therapist, and licensed professional counselor. A teacher turned therapist, she is now in private practice in Minneapolis and uses developmental movement therapy and somatic counseling to treat clients of all ages with symptoms of attention and learning challenges, including anxiety. In addition to her work with children and adults, Ms. Johnson is committed to educating new parents and care providers about the body's role in learning and the crucial role early movement has in optimal development. Stephanie lives in Minneapolis with her son. To learn more, visit babybare.net.